HEALTH AND HEALTH CARE

2010

THE FORECAST, THE CHALLENGE

CONTRIBUTORS

Authors: Roy Amara, Karen Bodenhorn, Mary Cain, Diana Cypress, Hank Dempsey, Wendy Everett, Rod Falcon, Roberto Garces, Matthew Holt, Susannah Kirsch, Heather Kuiper, Elaina Kyrouz, Robert Mittman, Ellen Morrison, Ian Morrison, Geoffrey Nilsen, Marina Pascali, Greg Schmid, Charlie Wilson, Kathy Yu

Editors: Charles Grosel, Melinda Hamilton, Julie Koyano, Susan Eastwood
Art Director: Janet Chambers
Graphic Designers: Adrianna Aranda, Robin Bogott, Diana Cypress, Jeanné Haffner, Melinda Hamilton

HEALTH AND HEALTH CARE

2010

THE FORECAST, THE CHALLENGE

Prepared by

The Institute for the Future

Support for this publication and conference was provided by

THE
ROBERT WOOD
JOHNSON
FOUNDATION

Princeton, NJ

January 2000

Jossey-Bass Publishers • San Francisco

Jossey-Bass books and products are available through most bookstores. To contact Jossey-Bass directly, call (888) 378-2537, fax to (800) 605-2665, or visit our website at www.josseybass.com.

Substantial discounts on bulk quantities of Jossey-Bass books are available to corporations, professional associations, and other organizations. For details and discount information, contact the special sales department at Jossey-Bass.

This book is printed on acid-free, recycled stock that meets or exceeds the minimum GPO and EPA requirements for recycled papers. Manufactured in the United States of America.

Library of Congress Cataloging-in-Publication Data

Health and health care 2010 : the forecast, the challenge / [contributors, Roy Amara . . . [et al.]]
     p. cm.
  "To recognize the 25th anniversary of its founding, The Robert Wood Johnson Foundation asked the Institute for the Future (IFTF) to forecast the future of health and and health care in America . . ."—Introduction.
  Includes bibliographical references and index.
  ISBN 0-7879-5348-2
    1. Medical care—United States—Forecasting. 2. Public Health—United States—Forecasting. I. Amara, Roy. II. Robert Wood Johnson Foundation. III Institute for the Future.

RA445 .H3364 2000
362.1'0973—dc21   99-088438

FIRST EDITION
PB Printing 10 9 8 7 6 5 4 3

HEALTH AND HEALTH CARE 2010

Contents

VI   Contents

FIGURES

TABLES

SIDEBARS

ABBREVIATIONS AND ACRONYMS

AAMC	American Association of Medical Colleges
AAPCC	adjusted average per capita costs
AARP	American Association of Retired Persons
AFDC	Aid to Families with Dependent Children
AHA	American Hospital Association
AIDS	acquired immunodeficiency syndrome
AMA	American Medical Association
AMC	academic medical center
CBO	Congressional Budget Office
CDC	Centers for Disease Control and Prevention
COGME	Council on Graduate Medical Education
CPR	computer-based patient record
CPS	Current Population Survey
CT	computed tomography
DRG	diagnosis-related group
DSH	disproportionate share hospital
EBRI	Employee Benefits Research Institute
EMR	electronic medical record
ETS	environmental tobacco smoke
FDA	Food and Drug Administration
FFS	fee for service
FTE	full-time equivalent
GDP	gross domestic product
GME	graduate medical education
HCFA	Health Care Financing Administration
HEDIS	health plan employer data and information set
HIPAA	Health Insurance Portability and Accountability Act
HIV	human immunodeficiency virus
HMO	health maintenance organization
HPV	human papilloma virus
IMGs	international medical graduates
IOM	Institute of Medicine

IPA	independent practice association
IVR	interactive voice response
LPN	licensed practical nurses
MRI	magnetic resonance imaging
MRN	magnetic resonance neurography
MSA	medical savings account
MSO	management services organization
MTBE	methlytertiary butyl ether
NAFTA	North American Free Trade Agreement
NCQA	National Committee on Quality Assurance
NHE	National Health Expenditure
NHIS	National Health Insurance Survey
NP	nurse practitioner
OTC	over the counter
PA	physician's assistant
PC	personal computer
PET	positron emission tomography
POS	point of service
PPM	physician practice management
PPO	preferred provider organization
PPS	prospective payment system
PSN	provider service network
RN	registered nurse
SAMHSA	Substance Abuse and Mental Health Services Association
SES	socioeconomic status
SIDS	sudden infant death syndrome
SNF	skilled nursing facility
SV40	simian virus 40
WHO	World Health Organization

HEALTH AND HEALTH CARE 2010

Introduction

To recognize the 25th anniversary of its founding, The Robert Wood Johnson Foundation asked the Institute for the Future (IFTF) to forecast the future of health and health care in America for the period between now and the year 2010. The purpose of this forecast is to provide the reader with a description of critical factors that will influence health and health care in the first decade of the 21st century.

In this book, we have singled out the trends most likely to influence the course of Americans' health and the state of the American health care delivery system between now and the year 2010. The drivers of this system are relatively stable and predictable from now to 2005. Beyond 2005, and through to 2010, the future of health and health care is much more volatile.

To cope with the uncertainties that exist for these later years, IFTF has created three different scenarios that describe emerging visions of health care in this country. They are titled Stormy Weather, The Long and Winding Road, and The Sunny Side of the Street, and they are described in the first chapter of this report. We hope that the findings of this study will be of value to community service organizations, hospitals, providers, payers, and researchers in the long-term planning processes that support their own visions of the future.

This forecast is organized in the following way:

- *Health and Health Care Forecast*
  This first chapter provides an overview of the important issues covered in greater detail throughout the forecast. It functions as an executive summary of the topics that are covered in greater detail in the subsequent chapters.

- *Demographic Trends and the Burden of Disease*
  In 2010, the American population will be older and more ethnically and racially diverse. The burden of disease is shifting toward chronic illnesses that stem from our behaviors. This chapter draws attention to the importance of these shifts.

- *Health Care's Demand Side*
  The growth rate of American health care costs steadily increased from 1960 through the early 1990s, then slowed dramatically. This chapter reviews the historical factors that drove these changes and forecasts the health care cost increases in both the public and private sectors over the next 10 years.

■ *Health Insurance*
Changes in the health insurance system and in the numbers of the uninsured are discussed in this chapter. The growth of Medicare and Medicaid, as well as new versions of managed care products, are projected through the year 2010.

■ *Health Care Providers*
There will be continued change in the way health care is organized and delivered over the next 10 to 15 years. The surplus of hospital beds will contribute to a buyer's market, and a new role for intermediaries will emerge. This chapter examines in depth the battle that will evolve in the medical management arena.

■ *Health Care Workforce*
There has been little real change in the way physicians practice medicine since the invention of the telephone. Although physicians are still the central figures in American health care, the current oversupply of doctors and the emergence of new health care provider roles may create changes in the health care delivery system over the next decade. The supply and demand of these providers are projected through 2010.

■ *Medical Technologies*
New medical technologies have been one of the key driving forces in both the cost and the organization of 20th-century health care. This chapter reviews eight new medical technologies that will affect the provision of patient care in the next 10 years and examines both their potential positive effects and the barriers that may stand in the way of their adoption.

■ *Information Technologies*
The health care industry has lagged behind other industries in implementing information technologies that streamline business and clinical processes. We forecast that changes in information technology as applied to health care will be a prime catalyst of change in the future.

■ *Health Care Consumers*
As a new, educated generation of informed consumers begins to use more health services, it is demanding more information, choice, and control than ever before. These empowered consumers have the capacity to change dramatically the culture of health care. In addition, the press of health care cost containment may lead to a three-tiered system of access to care that seriously disenfranchises people who do not have insurance.

■ *Public Health Services*
Modern public health is practiced in an environment of increasing globalism and resource scarcity. New developments in technology, public health strategy, and public-private partnerships will shape future successes and failures in public health. This chapter examines and forecasts the future of public health services, including organizational and environmental health issues.

■ *Health Behaviors*
Our health behaviors, namely smoking, poor dietary habits, lack of exercise, alcohol abuse, the use of illicit drugs, and violence, influence up to 50 percent of our health status. Although we do not anticipate radical improvements in these health behav-

iors in the coming decade, the emphasis that managed care has placed on prevention will help us begin to decrease these harmful behaviors. In addition, community-based programs that change or restrict the environment will also be very important.

- *Expanded Perspective on Health*
A definition of health must have equal applicability to everyone: to the fully well, to people who are unwell because of disease or illness that is treatable or curable, and to that growing segment of the population with genetic or acquired impairment, such as people with chronic disease or disability. Over the next decade, our view of health will be expanded to encompass mental, social, and spiritual well-being.

WILD CARDS

Wild cards are events that have less than a 10 percent chance of occurring, but will have a tremendous impact on society and business if they do occur. The point of wild cards is not to predict an outcome but to expand peripheral vision regarding the total range of possibilities; to offer a larger context within which to consider mainstream forecasts; and to prepare for surprises in the event they do come to pass.

ABOUT THE INSTITUTE FOR THE FUTURE

Located at the northern edge of Silicon Valley in Menlo Park, California, IFTF is an independent, nonprofit research firm that specializes in long-term forecasting. Founded in 1968, IFTF has become a leader in applied research for nonprofit organizations, corporations, industries,

and governments. IFTF has a cross-disciplinary professional staff that works internationally, analyzing policy, forecasting potential scenarios of the future, and identifying markets for new products and next-generation technologies.

IFTF's Health Team is in its 15th year of providing health care data tracking and forecasting based on primary research data. Our research projects focus on emerging trends in the organization, financing, and delivery of health care services, technologies, and products, with an emphasis on public policy changes as well as the impact of private sector markets. The Health Team evaluates the forces that both drive and resist innovation and forecasts not only the direction but also the pace of change in the health and health care environment.

ACKNOWLEDGMENTS

The idea for this study originated with Ruby Hearn, PhD, and Steven Schroeder, MD, of The Robert Wood Johnson Foundation. They believed that there would be value in developing the forecast as a long-range strategic planning tool for health organizations. Along with Dr. Hearn and Dr. Schroeder, Frank Karel, Beth Stevens, PhD, Ann Searight, Maureen Cozine, Nancy Kaufman, PhD, and Jeanne Weber provided consistent oversight and cogent direction to the project, helping all of us to focus, refine, and improve the final product. Lois Shevlin and Phyllis Kane were invaluable in guiding us through the planning and development processes. We are indebted to them and are extremely grateful for their support and guidance throughout this project.

The IFTF staff could not have completed the research necessary to formulate this forecast without the help of many colleagues, experts, and friends. Among those who were instrumental in identifying and refining issues and trends with us, we would like to thank particularly the following people:

Nancy Adler, PhD; Adrianna Aranda; Morris Barer, PhD; John Berthko; Katherine Binns; Bob Blendon, ScD; Robin Bogott; Janet Chambers; Toby Cole, MD; Rena Convissor; John Danaher, MD; Karen Davis, PhD; Joe DeLuca; Al Dembe; Susan Edgman-Levitan; Bob Evans, PhD; Michael Goldberg; Michael Goze; Peter Grant, Jessie Gruman, PhD; David Gustafson, PhD; Melinda Hamilton; David Hansen; Kathy Harty; David Hayes-Bautista, PhD; David Hemenway, PhD; Patrick Jeffries; Don Kemper; Bill Kerr; Quita Kirk; Paula Lack; Kim Lawrence; Julia Lear, PhD; Bob Leitman; Jeff Lemieux; Katherine Levit; Molly Mettler; Arnie Milstein, MD; Al Mulley, MD; Al Martin, MD; Gordon Moore, MD; H. Richard Nesson, MD; Mark Petrakis; James Robinson, PhD; Richard Rockefeller, MD; John Rother; Pamela Russell; Bill Scanlon; Monica Seghers; Cary Sennet, MD; J. J. Singh; Mark Smith, MD; Elliott Sternberg, MD; Felicia Stewart, MD; Jon Stewart; Humphrey Taylor; Sally Tom; Joan Trauner, PhD; and Leonard Zegans, MD.

Their thoughtfulness, insightful comments, and generous contributions of time and energy added significantly to our own knowledge and to the robustness of the forecast.

Special thanks go to Julie Koyano and Susan Eastwood for their sensational editorial work and patience, and to Andy Pasternack and Jon Peck for their guidance in publishing this work.

With thanks,

Wendy Everett
Director

Roy Amara

Mary Cain

Diana Cypress

Hank Dempsey

Rod Falcon

Danielle Gasper

Matthew Holt

Susannah Kirsch

Heather Kuiper

Elaina Kyrouz

Robert Mittman

Ellen Morrison

Ian Morrison

Geoffrey Nilsen

Marina Pascali

Denise Runde

Greg Schmid

Charlie Wilson

Kathy Yu

*Institute for the Future
Menlo Park, California*

Karen Bodenhorn

Roberto Garces

California Center for Health Improvement

HEALTH AND HEALTH CARE

2010

THE FORECAST, THE CHALLENGE

CHAPTER 1

Health and Health Care Forecast

Executive Summary

Ten years ago, the key issues in the American health care system were classic: containing *costs* while improving *access* to care for people and maintaining *quality* of services. Then the rapid cost increases of the late 1980s, combined with the recession of the early 1990s, added a new issue to the list: ensuring *security of benefits*.

After the political dust of the 1992–1994 debate about health reform settled, several structural shifts in the system became apparent. Managed care—designed to contain costs—went from being an aberration to being the mainstream method of providing health insurance. Several new issues came to the forefront of health policy: monitoring the activities of managed care plans, organizing health care providers, and evaluating the quality of care delivered to patients. Although the recent strong economy and job market has increased the security of health benefits for some people, the issue of how to pay for care for a growing number of uninsured Americans remains with us.

None of these issues will be completely resolved in the next 5 years. Instead, a new group of issues will join them. They include organizing insurers and intermediaries, along with providers; incorporating consumers into health care decision

making; determining responsibility for medical management; and improving the health behaviors of the American people. These will be the health battlegrounds of the next decade.

This chapter provides an overview of our 10-year forecast of health and health care. We describe the path from now until 2005 in terms of the future legislative and regulatory contexts; changes in the demographics and attitudes of patients, populations, and consumers; the concerns of payers about health care costs; the organization of health plans and insurers; the structure of hospitals, provider organizations, and the public health system; the role of medical information technologies; and the forthcoming shifts in care processes and medical management. Beyond 2005, our forecast splits into three scenarios—one optimistic about the impact of changes on the health of the population, one pessimistic about the ability of American society to provide coverage and access to care, and one in which incrementalism reigns supreme.

LEGISLATION

Legislative activity will be set against a background of incremental legislative reform. The failure of the health reform effort from 1992 to 1994 has dulled the appetite of most politicians for significant health regulation. In addition, there is almost no support for large-scale social programs targeting the poor or the uninsured. Major government reform is therefore unlikely. Strong support for the current Medicare and Social Security systems means that change in the benefits of these systems will be slow. There will be few initiatives to design new government programs beyond the limited programs enacted in the past few years—insurance portability and children's coverage. Neither of these two initiatives will have a significant impact on the overall number of uninsured or the general health insurance market.

Government legislation in two significant areas will have some impact on the mainstream health care system.

First, there will be legislative outcomes as a result of a backlash against managed care. While there are few clearly articulated alternatives to market-based health care in the United States, there is considerable support for legislation to curb what are seen as health plan abuses. Given that these regulations will require little money from public coffers, we can expect more regulation of health plan activity, including disclosure rules, mandates for clinical protocols such as the 48-hour hospital stay for maternity patients, and medical records privacy laws. Although the effect of such regulations on the overall market may be slight, there will be significant effects on plan and provider operations.

Second, Medicare may look very different than it did in the early 1990s, when its financial future became uncertain. Many Medicare recipients will not be in the traditional fee-for-service (FFS) program but instead will be in health maintenance organizations (HMOs), preferred provider organizations (PPOs), or some other organized health plan arrangement. Cost controls enacted in the 1997 Balanced Budget Act will have changed the way providers deal with Medicare patients, in particular placing the reimbursement for outpatient, home health, and skilled nursing facilities (SNFs) on a prospective payment system. It's plausible that the baseline will be sufficiently different that "incremental" legislation in the future could make a big change in the nature of the program. But Medicare remains the second most popular program among the most powerful demographic group in America—the elderly—and politicians have learned to tamper with it at their peril.

Consequently, our forecast for legislation is one of continued incremental program change directed primarily at providers and with little direct effect on beneficiaries. The real challenge—changing Medicare so that it can afford to cover the vast number of baby boomers retiring after 2010—will not be dealt with until later in the decade.

DEMOGRAPHICS: PATIENTS, POPULATIONS, AND NEW CONSUMERS

In the next decade, Americans will be getting older and living longer. By 2010 the average life expectancy will be up to

Figure 1-1. Increasing Diversity of the United States Population

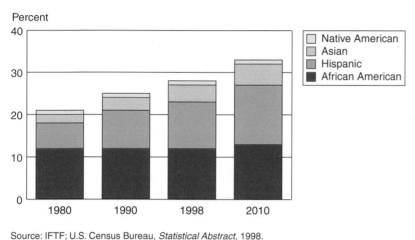

Source: IFTF; U.S. Census Bureau, *Statistical Abstract*, 1998.

Figure 1-2. The Real Story of Diversity Is Regional in 2010

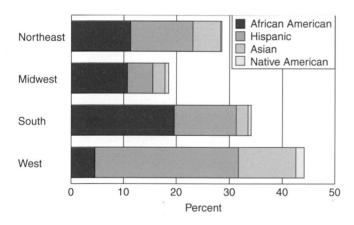

Source: IFTF; U.S. Census Bureau.

Tiers of Coverage

Empowered Consumers:	38 percent
Worried Consumers:	34 percent
Excluded Consumers:	28 percent

86 years of age for a woman and 76 years for a man. In addition, there will be more than 100,000 people over the age of 100 in the year 2010. However, the first baby boomers will not turn 65 until 2010, so although the population is aging, it's aging quite slowly.

America will soon be a more ethnically diverse nation (see Figures 1-1 and 1-2). Currently 74 percent of the population is white, but that will decrease to about 64 percent by the year 2010. Asians will make up 5 percent, and African Americans 13 percent. In the more densely populated western states, approximately 15 percent of the population will be Hispanic.

The population will also be better educated in 2005: 55 percent of the population age 25 years and older will have the equivalent of one year of college (see Figure 1-3). Income disparity—a critical factor in determining health—will increase slightly. In the year 2005, 50 percent of the population will have a family income of $53,000 or more in constant 1998 dollars, and the distribution will be slightly more equal.

Access to care will remain "tiered" and that tiering will become much more extreme. The top tier, the "empowered consumers," have considerable discretionary income, are well educated, and use technology (including the Internet) to get information about their health. These new consumers increasingly will engage in shared decision making with their physicians.

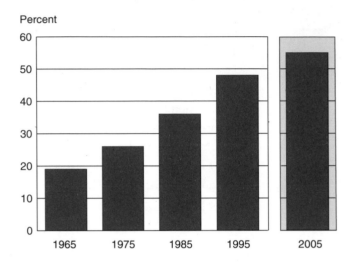

Figure 1-3. A Growing Number of Adults in the United States Have Attended College (Percentage of people age 25 years and older who have attended college).

Percent

Source: U.S. Census Bureau.

PAYERS AND HEALTH CARE COSTS

The health care system has been dominated by cost concerns for the better part of 30 years, but that domination will wane during the next decade. From 1965 to 1991—from the inception of Medicare and Medicaid through the recession that precipitated the Great Health Care Reform Debate of 1992—health care grew from 5 percent of the gross domestic product (GDP) to more than 13 percent. It is now at about 14 percent of GDP, with virtually all the reduction in cost growth coming from savings in the private sector.

We forecast a moderate but consistent increase in the cost of health care between now and 2005. Health care will grow as a share of the economy,[1] albeit more slowly than in the 1960s, 1970s, and 1980s. By 2005, the health care sector will account for about 15 percent of GDP. Employers in the private sector will see the short-lived cost decreases of the mid-1990s fade away.[2] They'll see nominal cost increases of 3 to 6 percent per year. Despite the best efforts of Congress to reduce spending in the Medicare system, public programs will continue to grow between 6 and 9 percent per year.

Between now and 2005, business and government will put several strategies in place to repress large cost increases. These strategies tend to assuage the symptoms rather than to attack the cause of the increases. The strategies include reducing insurance coverage, passing on the costs of health care premiums to beneficiaries, and increasing the restrictions on access to care via financial disincentives for utilization.

The second tier is made up of the "worried consumers." These are consumers who have access to some health insurance but have little or no choice of health plans. This tier includes those whose employers only offer one type of coverage and those who may be temporarily employed and face an even less secure health insurance outlook. This "worried" group also includes early retirees and others who do not have the same access to discretionary income as the empowered consumers.

The third tier is composed of the "excluded consumers." In this group are the uninsured, people on Medicaid, and others who don't have access to market-based health insurance. Throughout our forecast, these three groups are affected in varying ways by different aspects of the health care system.

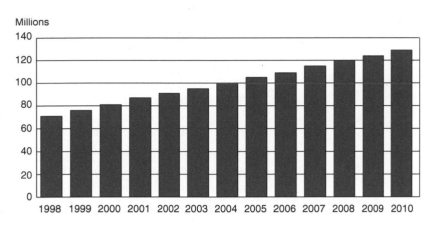

Figure 1-4. Americans Move into HMOs

Millions

Source: Group Health Administration of America, Interstudy, American Association of Health Plans.

The health insurance market will evolve into a mix of different health plan models, many of which will spend the next several years in a constant flurry of reorganization and mergers. Four dominant "intermediary" models will emerge by 2005: the case manager, the provider partner, the high-end FFS broker, and the safety-net funder. As a result, in 2007 close to 50 percent of the population will be in health plans for which cost containment is a key issue.

Despite all the pressures toward increasing costs in the system, these new strategies will be successful enough to keep costs from exploding again as they did from 1960 to 1990.

HEALTH PLANS AND INSURERS

The biggest change in the health insurance market over the past 10 years has been the fast growth of HMO enrollment. In 1998, more than 78 million Americans were enrolled in HMOs, and a majority were in some kind of a managed care plan. By 2005, HMOs will capture the majority of the commercial market and more than 25 percent of the Medicare market. Sixty percent of Medicaid recipients will be in some form of HMO by the year 2010.[3]

Among this plethora of new products, it will be increasingly difficult to distinguish one health plan from another. They'll all offer similar—and often the same—providers and pay those providers through a mixture of discounted FFS and capitation. By 2005, more than 100 million people will be in these "HMO descendants." (See Figure 1-4.)

HOSPITALS AND PHYSICIANS

As the demand side evolves, changes in the ways providers are organized will occur in the context of significant provider oversupply (see Figure 1-5). There are 570,000 physicians in the United States and another 170,000 in the medical school pipeline. There are nearly three new physicians for every one doctor who retires. Moreover, the numbers of nurse practitioners (NPs), physician's assistants (PAs), and other non-MD clinicians will increase rapidly over the next decade. Physicians are moving into group practices, yet it will be 2005 before most office-based physicians are in groups, and most of those will be in groups of six or fewer.

On the hospital side, occupancy percentage rates have fallen from the low 80s to the low 60s in the past decade, but neither beds nor hospitals have closed at a

Total supply of nonfederal
patient-care physicians

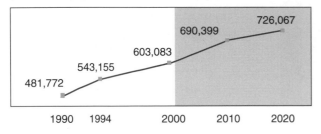

Nonfederal patient-care physicians
per 100,000 civilian population

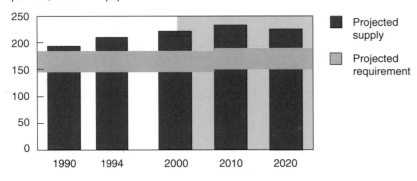

Source: IFTF; Bureau of Health Professions, American Medical Association, Council on Graduate Medical Education.

interventions of health plans that have driven much activity out of the inpatient setting will continue, but at a relatively slower pace.

MEDICAL AND INFORMATION TECHNOLOGIES

Technological change is accelerating in two areas that will affect health care dramatically: medical and information technologies. Medical technology has been one of the major drivers of the health care system since the introduction of effective pharmacological agents in the early part of this century. Its impact will continue in the next decade. However, health care has not made significant use of the advances in information technology that have transformed most other industries. That situation will not continue for much longer as the boundaries between information and medical technologies begin to blur.

MEDICAL TECHNOLOGIES

The health care system has quickly adopted new medical technologies, both devices and pharmaceuticals. Despite increased interest in cost-benefit assessment techniques, the pace of introducing new technologies is unlikely to slow, and there will be a significant increase in the number of new technologies available in the coming decade. Some of the most interesting new technologies include:

- *Rational drug design*. The use of computers to design drugs that target a particular receptor.

- *Advances in imaging*. The use of new imaging technologies—such as

rate that's close to the drop in demand. Set against this background of institutional inertia, no dominant model will emerge to replace the large teaching hospital and smaller community hospital models that provided medical care from the 1930s to the early 1990s.

There will be some hospital closings and bed reductions, but hospitals will continue to be difficult to shut down. From a total of just over 850,000 beds in 1997, we anticipate a further reduction of 130,000 beds by 2005.[4] The advances in medical technology and the aggressive electron-beam computed tomography (CT), harmonic ultrasound, high-resolution positron emission tomography (PET), and functional magnetic resonance imaging (MRI)—to look at the form and function of organs that were once examined only in surgery.

- *Minimally invasive surgery.* The use of miniaturized devices, digitized imaging, and vascular catheters in neurosurgery, cardiology, and interventional radiology.

- *Genetic mapping and testing.* The identification and testing of genes and genetic interactions that cause disease.

- *Gene therapy.* The use of site-specific genes to treat a variety of inherited or acquired diseases.

- *Vaccines.* The use of vaccines to bolster immune systems, target tumors, or immunize against viruses, and of delivery methods including oral and nasal sprays to simplify the vaccination processes.

- *Artificial blood.* The use of recombinant hemoglobin, using *E. coli,* to create a blood substitute.

- *Xenotransplantation.* The transplantation of tissues and organs from animals into humans, primarily bone marrow and solid organs.

INFORMATION TECHNOLOGIES

The information and communications revolution will move into the health care system in the next 7 to 12 years. We forecast that four main areas will be affected by new information technologies and that

together they'll be the drivers behind new clinical care processes. They are:

- *Automation of basic business processes.* The transaction standards mandated in the 1996 Health Insurance Portability and Accountability Act (HIPAA) legislation will move plans and providers toward automation of the submission and adjudication of claims, determination of patient eligibility, coordination of benefits, and authorizations of referrals beginning early in the year 2000.

- *Clinical information interfaces.* The creation of an electronic medical record (EMR) has stumbled because of resistance from providers, even while many of the basic building blocks are being put into place. Over the next decade, the availability of computers, sophisticated decision support systems, and voice recognition will create interfaces that are clinician-friendly. A combination of low equipment prices, younger, computer-savvy clinicians, and the move of physicians into groups will cause a slow but certain adoption of computerized medical records in the years after 2005.

- *Data analysis.* In the next few years, administrative and claims data sets will be extensively "mined" to gain a better understanding of a population's future illnesses and an improved ability to risk-adjust payments to health plans and providers. After 2005, there will be more data available directly from clinical records. There will be close to real-time online analytical processing of information about patient and provider outcomes, and that information will be used in all aspects of health care.

- *Telehealth.* A combination of computer-supported case management, remote telemetry via sensors, and better-informed patients will create new ways of delivering health care. Chronically ill patients will be monitored remotely by using a variety of sensor devices, such as video cameras, blood pressure monitors, blood glucose readers, and smart pill boxes. Sensors will be linked to computer systems that enable the provider to catch adverse events almost before they happen. The vast increase in information about health that the Internet, interactive TV, and other communications media bring into the home will also affect the health care system. Patients will use these media for disease-specific research, psychosocial support groups, self-care, and shared decision making.

We forecast that the impact of medical technologies on the health care system will continue to be significant, although the true gains from using information technology and computerizing clinical care processes will not be seen until after 2005.

CARE PROCESSES AND MEDICAL MANAGEMENT

Medical management—the active management of the care of patients and populations—is currently applied sporadically, if at all. There are two main issues in the future of medical management. The first is the debate over which care processes are used. Many groups are developing guidelines and practice protocols, but none has agreed how, where, or when to use them. The second is the need to reduce variations in practice, thereby reducing costs and improving clinical outcomes. Since an individual clinician is less able to judge adherence to protocols than is a manager reviewing records of an entire organization, decisions about medical management will continue to shift away from the prerogative of the independent physician. Instead, internal managers in provider organizations and external managers working for intermediaries and plans will assume increasing authority in managing physicians' behavior and patients' compliance. Because medical management will depend on information systems to monitor and track both processes and outcomes, we forecast that putting these medical management processes in place will take closer to 15 years than 5 years.

In the interim, disease and demand management programs for the well population—advice nurses working with patients using the telephone and the Internet—will be commonplace. The advent of disease management programs and the adoption of clinical guidelines will have a significant impact on medical practice and patient management by 2005 and a sporadic but discernible effect on practice variation a few years later. However, the struggle between intermediaries and providers and among different provider organizations over who controls patients' and physicians' behavior will not be resolved by 2010.

PUBLIC HEALTH

Over the past 30 years the public health system has operated under pressures of resource scarcity, limits in leadership, and organizational fragmentation. As the public health system assumed the role of safety-net medical provider, the economic burden upon it became almost unbearable. Public health also suffered an identity crisis as the public confused public health with indigent medical care, further diminishing support for a population-based health infrastructure. At the same time, new health challenges emerged, such as HIV/AIDS and environmental contamination, that required strong leadership and an integration of population-based approaches into public health.

Overarching global forces will determine the context in which public health functions in the future. Ten years from now the currently inchoate social vision reshaping government will have fully emerged and will determine the players and resources in future public health leadership and action. Furthermore, global economies and populations will drive increases in health risks, and by the next decade, national public health concerns will be embedded in a global context of threats and opportunities. Cost-effective technological advances, while mitigated by ethical debate, will enhance screening, surveillance, and environmental health. Finally, public health will increasingly employ "ecological" strategies that simultaneously address multiple human and structural determinants of health and health behavior.

During most of the next decade, public health will continue to be underfunded and marginalized, and efforts to address these underlying problems will be largely incremental. Breaches in public health prevention systems will become increasingly evident, but the system will not

totally collapse because support for public health will increase enough to maintain at least a minimal system. The rise of the new consumer will also increase support for public health measures.

Over the next decade, national public health policy will be generally piecemeal, but dynamic state-level actions will generate enough momentum to reignite federal comprehensive health care reform debate. Community coalitions that assure access to basic personal and public health services will become more common. Managed care will continue to dominate, but will be augmented by the integration of population and personal health, public and private patient bases, and a variety of reimbursement strategies. The full potency, limitations, and consequences of public health litigation, à la tobacco, also will be evident in the next decade.

The future of public health service delivery will be shared among the local public health agencies, the community's private health care providers and organizations, and community-based organizations and leaders. The science of epidemiology will continue to be one of public health's most useful guides and will extend beyond biomedical applications to evaluate innovative and comprehensive public health prevention strategies.

Tobacco use will continue its steady decline, but at a very slow pace. In some geographic regions, use may remain at the current plateau. Community-based actions and local legislation will remain effective tactics in curbing tobacco use in public places. A persistent influx of youth smokers will require constant vigilance,

Forecast Through 2005

Health Care Spending Growth:	2 percent per year above nominal GDP growth
Health Care Spending:	15 percent of GDP, $6,424 per capita
Uninsurance Rate:	44 million uninsured, 15 percent of population

especially as smoking interacts with alcohol and illicit drug use. Abuse of these substances, in the absence of significant augmentation of treatment and prevention programs, will continue to fluctuate at high but not record-breaking levels. Barring a massive economic recession, firearm injuries related to violence will continue their already 5-year decline, with slower declines in nonviolent firearm injury gaining momentum as an array of interventions take effect. Although levels of infectious disease in the early 21st century will not approximate those of the early 20th century, (re)emerging infections, drug resistance, resurgence in risky behaviors, threats of bioterrorism, and the interaction of infec-

What Level of Health Care Spending Growth Is Sustainable in the Long Run?

A sea change in health care spending took place in the early 1990s. The annual growth rate dropped from 11 percent—a rate that had been sustained since the 1960s—to 6.75 percent. A combination of forces converged to lower spending growth: strong price pressure from employer coalitions and other large purchasers; a low point in the health insurance underwriting cycle; and providers' and suppliers' keeping their prices in check during the health reform debate and its aftermath. A key question for the next 10 years is this: Do we sustain the recent, 5-year pattern of low growth rates in spending or do we return to the historical, 30-year pattern of higher growth? Scenario One reflects the 30-year pattern of spending growth. Scenarios Two and Three reflect the more recent 5-year pattern of spending growth.

tious and chronic disease will keep infectious diseases on the public health attention list. Finally, the by-products of our modern society will gain markedly increased attention in the next decade as food safety and air and water quality reach critical points. The crucible for environmental health action will be child health and safety actions and standards.

THREE SCENARIOS

Our forecast is relatively certain and stable through the year 2005. Beyond 2005, we have created three scenarios to describe how the health care landscape might evolve.

SCENARIO ONE: STORMY WEATHER

In the Stormy Weather scenario, pressures from rising costs, dissatisfied providers and patients, marked inequality of access to care, greedy profit takers, and repeated health care scandals accumulate through the year 2005. None of the fundamental problems of cost, quality, or access are addressed in a meaningful way. Between 2005 and 2010, the barometer drops, winds converge, and stormy weather erupts. The primary driving forces in this scenario include:

- Managed care programs that fail to deliver on their promises to contain costs or to improve quality. Instead, they default to more hassling of providers and gaming of utilization management systems.

- Consumers and providers who react to the adversarial climate with a strong, unified backlash to managed care. They succeed in getting legislation

Scenario One Indicators

Health Care Spending Growth:	2.5 percent per year above nominal GDP growth
Health Care Spending:	19 percent of GDP, $10,200 per capita
Uninsurance Rate:	65 million uninsured, 22 percent of population

passed that further erodes the effectiveness of managed care by intervening in a variety of clinical and structural decisions, such as regulation of lengths of stay for various procedures, staffing ratios, and any-willing-provider laws.

■ Health plans that engage in substantial adverse selection and cream-skimming of beneficiaries as Medicare moves toward managed care and a wider range of choices for its beneficiaries. Medicare risk plans manage to get the bulk of low-cost, healthy beneficiaries, leaving the sick, costly people to the conventional indemnity plan. Each attempt at risk adjustment is met with strategies that boost overall Medicare spending.

■ Provider oligopolies, including large group practices, physician practice management firms, national single-specialty groups, and large hospital chains, that are able to sustain high prices in an environment that demands open provider networks. They threaten to leave the networks of plans that don't pay well and the plans blink first.

■ Large employers that continue to offer insurance as a benefit of employment in the face of a tight labor market and are unable to demand substantial price breaks from health plans. Many small employers, meanwhile, drop insurance benefits altogether, substantially increasing the number of uninsured.

■ The march of new medical technologies, which continues unabated. Consumers, prompted both by pharmaceutical companies' direct-to-consumer advertising and by "gee-whiz" articles in the popular press, demand access to the latest, greatest, and most expensive drugs and medical technologies. Beleaguered health plans concede the point and lose control over cost and quality.

■ Costly medical technologies for extending life that are not restricted, as no social consensus develops to limit spending on health care near the end of life.

■ Information technologies, once thought to be the way to efficiency, consistency, and higher-quality care, that will prove to be costly and ineffective. Plans and providers find that their investments in the late 1990s and early 2000s don't pay off, but seeing no better way, they continue to invest after 2005.

■ The public health system, which will be in tatters, with local public health departments retreating from service provision and only minimally fulfilling mandated functions, and no compensatory response from the private sector.

Scenario One plays out with a range of difficult consequences. Health care spending, by 2010, constitutes almost one-fifth of gross domestic spending. Even with expenditures at that level,

Chapter 1: Health and Health Care Forecast   11

more than one in five Americans remains uninsured. A majority worry about losing their health benefits. Insecurity of benefits is widespread as many people are just one job change away from being without health insurance. Even those who retain insurance are a lot less happy as their out-of-pocket costs rise.

The health system exhibits radical tiering, with much poorer access to care for the uninsured and people on Medicaid. Medicaid itself puts enormous strain on states, as the state programs are faced with medical costs that overwhelm recession-depleted state budgets. A number of major public hospitals are forced to close their doors. Although their closing helps bring the supply of hospital beds into closer relation to the demand, it also strands many people who have nowhere else to go. The Medicare program finds itself unprepared to absorb the baby boomers, who begin to become eligible in 2010. By the end of the forecast period, health reform is again on the public policy agenda.

SCENARIO TWO: THE LONG AND WINDING ROAD

In Scenario Two, The Long and Winding Road, incrementalism reigns. The successive attempts at revising a portion of the health care system work sufficiently well that tinkering continues well past 2005. As costs get pushed down in one place, they pop up in another, but the system is able to respond rapidly and keep costs in balance. The primary driving forces for this scenario include:

- Employers who continue to pay close attention to health care costs and their benefit structures. They keep substantial price pressure on health plans, limiting increases on the commercial side to 3 to 4 percent per year. They also shift cost and risk to employees by moving increasingly from a defined benefit plan to a defined contribution program. As beneficiaries' out-of-pocket costs increase, utilization of health care services drops off in response.

- Health plans that, in turn, increase pressure on providers. They convince employers that they can only control utilization in a more closed network, so the expansive networks of the late 1990s disappear. In their place are more tightly controlled networks that exert both clinical control and strong price pressure on providers.

- Providers who—stung by the high cost and organizational difficulty of forming large units and integrating care—adopt few of the innovations of the leading-edge provider groups. Instead, they engage in sustained, and largely unsuccessful, resistance to being "hassled" by insurers.

- The cost-containment provisions of the 1998 federal budget, which rein in both Medicare and Medicaid spending. The provisions stick. That bill sets the standard for budget bills for the first 10 years of the next century.

- The public health system, which will engage in the dynamic competition with the private sector in service delivery.

The period of 2005 through 2010 is one of turbulent, disorganized change. The health care landscape changes as much in

Scenario Two Indicators

Health Care Spending Growth: 1 to 2 percent per year above nominal GDP growth

Health Care Spending: 16 percent of GDP, $8,600 per capita

Uninsurance Rate: 47 million uninsured, 16 percent of population

those 5 years as it did in the period from 1993 to 1998.

In Scenario Two, costs grow only a little faster than nominal GDP growth, reaching 16 percent of GDP by 2010. Federal and commercial cost containment work well enough to make insurance coverage affordable for most employers. About one in six Americans (47 million) is uninsured.

The health care system remains tiered, with about 20 percent of Americans in the bottom tier of public coverage and uninsurance, 60 percent in managed care plans that substantially restrict their choice of providers and limit providers' autonomy, and 20 percent in high-end, indemnity-type programs.

The bottom tier safety-net providers face tighter conditions, with cuts in disproportionate share hospital (DSH) funding, an end to cost-based reimbursement for outpatient clinics, and tight state and local budgets. But they manage to muddle through as usual by patching together a range of disparate funding sources.

Care delivery is still fragmented, as national players remain relatively rare and small. The majority of physicians now practice in groups of three or more,

but most of those are in three- to six-doctor groups. These groups are not large enough to accept global capitation safely, align with a hospital, or influence their physicians' practice patterns radically.

Comprehensive health reform does not enter the public policy debate, as incremental changes each year reassure elected officials that they are "doing something about health care."

SCENARIO THREE: THE SUNNY SIDE OF THE STREET

In the Sunny Side of the Street scenario, all the hard work and investment from now until 2005 pays off after 2005 in the form of a sustainable, efficient health care system. Competition helps drive excess capacity out of the system. We learn what does and does not work in medicine, and especially how to get providers and patients to work effectively together. Health plans and providers put in place information and management systems that can take the health care system through the next 2 decades. The driving forces for this scenario include:

- Competition at all levels of the health care system, but especially among providers, which helps drive costs down. Young physicians enter the market with lower income expectations and more of an employee mentality than their predecessors.

- The wave of consolidation of the late 1990s, which continues through the early 2000s. Efficient health care organizations, which can assimilate the best practices from their constituent parts, emerge. Consolidation also

Chapter 1: Health and Health Care Forecast

Scenario Three Indicators

Health Care Spending Growth:	1 percent per year above nominal GDP growth
Health Care Spending:	15 percent of GDP, $8,100 per capita
Uninsurance Rate:	30 million uninsured, 10 percent of population

serves to drive some excess capacity, especially of hospital beds although not necessarily hospitals themselves, out of the system.

- The provider service networks (PSNs) that form to contract with Medicare. PSNs find that they have efficient administrative structures. They begin to contract directly with employers in certain parts of the country. Medicare encourages further growth in its risk contracting as it develops effective risk-adjustment methods that make risk contracting cost-neutral for the program.

- Innovative payment approaches that are developed throughout the health care system. Prospective payment for outpatient services is put in place first by Medicare, then by commercial health plans.

- Health care information systems, which make significant progress beyond their current administrative functions. Clinical information systems are put in place that successfully improve care processes and outcomes. The EMR sees the light of day.

- Developments in medical technology that focus both on improving outcomes and on reducing costs. Regulators favor technologies that can demonstrate their cost-effectiveness as well as their safety and efficacy with more rapid approvals. Health plans and providers, through their improved information systems, develop the capacity to make trade-offs among therapies according to their cost-effectiveness.

- The public health sector, which will embrace public-private community partnerships, where service delivery occurs in the private sector and government focuses on assessment, development, and assurance.

In Scenario Three, cost growth is also just 1 percent above the nominal growth of GDP. By 2010, it reaches 15 percent of GDP. These moderate cost increases make health insurance more affordable. People experience more security of benefits, leaving an uninsurance rate of 10 percent (30 million people).

The good news is that the basics are in place—health systems are equipped to minimize unnecessary variation in practices, they operate efficiently, they can track what they're doing. The time spent cultivating a well-organized health system pays off in the long run. The bad news is that we still have 30 million people who are uninsured.

Medicare and private plans begin thinking about the long term. They put in place incentives to reward population management in addition to individual patient care. They also provide incentives for a longer-term focus on today's health care decisions. The system appears well equipped to take on the wave of baby boomers who will begin to be eligible for Medicare starting in 2010.

ENDNOTES

[1] We forecast that, during the next decade, real economic growth will remain at 2.5 percent, with general inflation in the economy averaging 3 percent. Health care cost growth at 5.5 percent will mean no change in the share of GDP going to health care. Faster growth of health care costs will mean that health care will grow as a share of GDP.

[2] Overall private sector cost increases averaged 4.8 percent from 1991 to 1995, but many large employers extracted actual premium decreases from health plans in a string of "famous victories" between 1993 and 1997.

[3] These 60 percent will account for only 30 percent of the costs of the program, as the blind, disabled, and dual-eligible elderly will still consume most of the resources.

[4] This doesn't tell the whole story as beds are often allocated to SNFs, 23-hour beds, or long-term care without moving from the same facility, but this projection is based on the official American Hospital Association (AHA) data for inpatient beds.

CHAPTER 2

Demographic Trends and the Burden of Disease

Increasing Diversity

Demographic shifts will shape the future. An increasing number of debates and discussions are surfacing around the social, economic, and health implications of demographic and social change. All of these concerns present new challenges for public policy, government, business, and the health care industry. Several critical issues and trends deserve attention—the aging baby boomers, the increasing ethnic and racial diversity, the growing disparity between the richest and the poorest households, and the future burden of disease.

This chapter examines each of these issues and sets the broad demographic context for examining the future of health and health care in America.

THE UNITED STATES POPULATION IS GROWING OLDER AND LIVING LONGER

The United States population is growing older—a demographic trend that will have far-reaching effects as the baby boom generation—those Americans born between 1946 and 1964—ages (see Figure 2-1). People 65 years of age and older

are the fastest-growing segment of the population. Their numbers will increase from 34 million in 1995 to 39 million in 2010, a 15 percent increase (see Figure 2-2). This "age wave" will have a transformational impact across many institutions, levels of government, and segments of society. The health care industry should begin planning now—well before 2010—to respond adequately to the needs of an older American population. The average life expectancy has increased by more than 30 years in this century and will be 86 for women and 76 for men in the year 2010 (see Figure 2-3).

The health care industry will certainly feel the effects of this demographic change in the next decade. Baby boomers have transformed many institutions and aspects of society along their life cycle— including the workplace, financial institutions, and government. As baby boomers interact with the health care system, their expectations and preferences will also transform these institutions as the health care industry adapts to accommodate baby boomers' demands and numbers. They will access the system not only for themselves but also for their parents and children. Boomers' involvement

Figure 2-1. America's Baby Boomers Are Aging

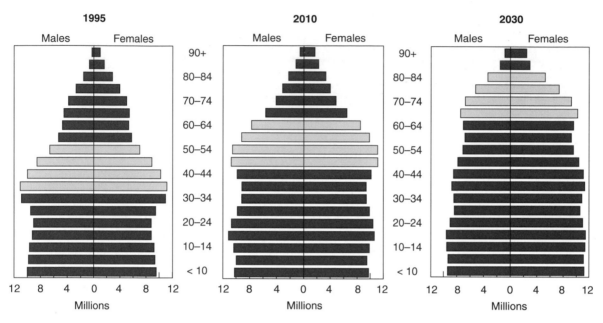

1995

Males | Females

2010

Males | Females

2030

Males | Females

Age groups (top to bottom): 90+, 80–84, 70–74, 60–64, 50–54, 40–44, 30–34, 20–24, 10–14, < 10

Axis (each chart): 12 8 4 0 4 8 12

Millions

Source: U.S. Census Bureau.

Figure 2-2. The Coming Surge in the Population of Age 65 Years and Older

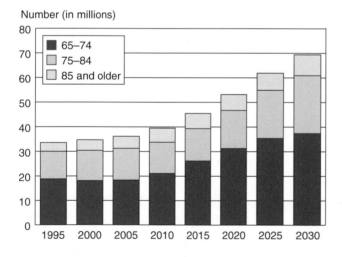

Number (in millions)

Legend:
- 65–74
- 75–84
- 85 and older

Axis: 0 10 20 30 40 50 60 70 80

Years: 1995 2000 2005 2010 2015 2020 2025 2030

Source: IFTF; U.S. Census Bureau.

in their own care will be distinctly different from that of past generations of older Americans. They will accelerate the movement and awareness of self-care and wellness and will irreversibly alter the traditional doctor–patient relationship (see Chapter 9).

However, the full impact of the aging population will not be felt until well after 2010, when baby boomers reach retirement age. Many baby boomers will enjoy better health and longer lives due in part to advances in health and medical technologies (see Chapter 7). With increasing longevity, boomers will lead more active and productive lives rather than simply retiring in old age, illustrating just one of the many social changes associated with this demographic shift.

Not until 2030, when the youngest baby boomer has reached the age of 65 and the entire baby boom's health care is subsidized by Medicare, will the nation's health and welfare system feel the true social and economic impact of this large age cohort. This trend signals the urgent need to resolve the problems of financing and delivering health care, social services, and long-term care for the population, as well as managing the health and health behaviors of this group.

THE FACE OF AMERICA CONTINUES TO CHANGE—DIVERSITY IS INCREASING

The United States is growing increasingly diverse. Although the population remains largely white non-Hispanic (73 percent), the Hispanic, African American, Asian, and Native American populations are all growing faster than the population as a whole—a trend driven by both higher immigration and higher birthrates among these groups. By 2010, minority ethnic and racial groups will account for 32 percent of the population, up from 20 percent in 1980. Yet the absolute number of ethnic and racial minorities will remain small and will continue to account for less than 50 percent of the population until well after 2050 (see Figure 2-4).

However, national data do not tell the full story—the real story of diversity is regional.

Hispanic, African American, Asian, and Native American populations are not evenly distributed across the United

Figure 2-3. Life Expectancy at Age 65 Has Increased Throughout the 20th Century, United States

Years of life remaining

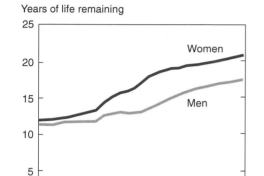

Source: Economic Report of the President, February 1999.

Figure 2-4. Increasing Diversity of the United States Population

Percent

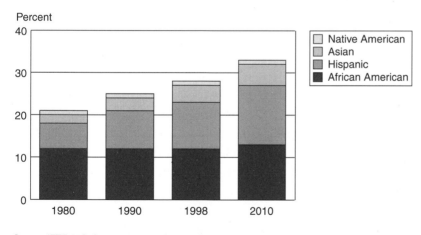

Source: IFTF; U.S. Census Bureau, *Statistical Abstract*, 1998.

States, making the issue of diversity more pronounced in certain regions than in others. Although the degree of diversity is increasing throughout the United States, the highest concentration of ethnic and racial minorities is found in the West, followed by the South, the Northeast, and the Midwest—a pattern that will continue (see Figure 2-5). In 2010, the concentration of African Americans will be highest in the South. The West will continue to be the most diverse multiethnic and multiracial region of the United States with the largest concentration of Hispanic, Asian, and Native American populations.

In addition to examining this issue at the regional level, it is important to look at specific states and metropolitan areas—a level where demographic profiles have more strategic meaning to health care providers. California, Illinois, New York, Florida, and Texas are all states where the issues of diversity are being confronted now. For example, in California, the Hispanic, Asian, African American, and Native American populations already account for 48 percent of the population—by 2010 no one ethnic or racial group (including whites) will be in the majority (see Figure 2-6). In cities such as Los Angeles, where 44 percent of the population is Hispanic, clinical providers are already facing the challenges of delivering care to a diverse population.

The increasing diversity of the population will place new demands on the health care industry. As the patient profile shows increasing proportions of Hispanic, African American, Asian, and Native American patients, the demand will become more pronounced for services that are culturally appropriate, beyond simple language competency. The concept of culturally appropriate services includes awareness of the complex issues related to the underdiagnosis of certain conditions and diseases among minority groups, the effects of lifestyle and cultural differences on health status, the implications of the diverse genetic endowment of the population, and the impact of patterns of assimilation on health status.

HOUSEHOLD INCOME IS INCREASING, BUT THE GAP BETWEEN THE EXTREMES IS WIDENING

Another key demographic shift is the growing number of households with high incomes. This trend is particularly important to consider in examining the future of both health and health care

Figure 2-5. The Real Story of Diversity Is Regional in 2010

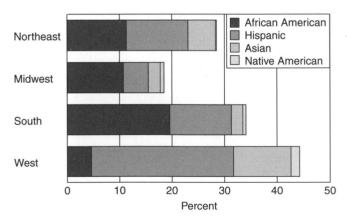

Source: IFTF; U.S. Census Bureau.

Chapter 2: Demographic Trends and the Burden of Disease

because income is related to both health status and access to health care services. Although various demographic characteristics are correlated with differences in health status, none is more highly correlated than income.

The recent boom in the United States economy has resulted in extraordinarily low unemployment rates, low inflation, high productivity, and a generally favorable economic outlook. This path of economic growth (2.5 percent in real terms) will lead to a longer-term sustainable expansion and will move many people into higher household income brackets. Households with higher incomes have higher levels of discretionary income and have better health status and access to care.

An examination of income distribution in the United States from 1970 to 2010 shows two significant trends emerging. First, the average per capita income in America will increase in real dollars. The good news is that higher income is associated with improved health status.[1] By 2010, the number of households with an income of $50,000 or more will reach 48 million, or 52 percent of all households—a number that is driven by the large number of baby boomers who will be well into their peak earning years (see Figure 2-7).

However, the pattern of income distribution reveals a second, more disturbing trend: a widening of the gap between the richest 25 percent and the poorest 25 percent of the population (see Figure 2-8). The prosperity of the 1980s and 1990s has moved many middle-class households into higher income tiers. By 2010, this pattern will be even more pronounced. Research has also shown that when income disparity among the population widens, the overall health status of the population worsens.[2] This projected income disparity will have negative consequences on the nation's overall health status and will remain a significant social and health issue well into the future.

Figure 2-6. California Is Ahead of the Nation

Percent

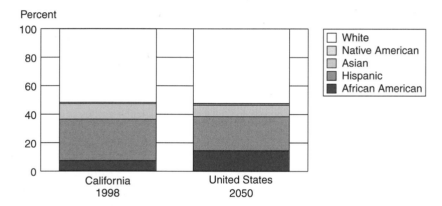

Source: IFTF; State of California, Department of Finance; U.S. Census Bureau.

Figure 2-7. The Number of Households Earning High Incomes Is Increasing

Percent

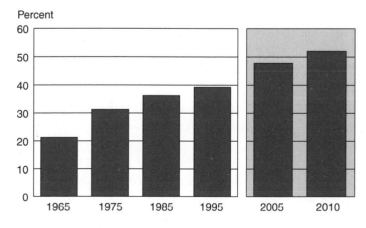

Source: IFTF; U.S. Census Bureau.

Figure 2-8. Redistribution of Income
(Percent of households by income in thousands of 1995 dollars)

100+			
90–100			
80–90			
70–80			
60–70			
50–60			
40–50			
30–40			
20–30			
10–20			
Under 10			
The Cathedral	The Bottle	The Vase	

Source: U.S. Census Bureau. *Money Income in the United States.* Current Population Survey, 1994.

THE SHIFTING BURDEN OF DISEASE: CHRONIC DISEASES, MENTAL ILLNESS, AND LIFESTYLE BEHAVIORS

In reviewing disease prevalence and causes of death over the past century, it is impossible to ignore the significant decrease in, and even eradication of, many infectious diseases. Vaccines, antibiotics, and biotechnological advances have curbed the communicable diseases of the 20th century. Simultaneously, there has been an increase in the incidence of chronic diseases, such as cancer and cardiovascular disease. One reason for this increase is the greater life expectancy enjoyed by many Americans. Many chronic illnesses, such as cardiovascular disease, generally strike people in their later years. Increases in life ex-

pectancy and in the proportion of elderly people are accompanied by an increased prevalence of chronic diseases. Although new medical innovations promise to make a dent in the prevalence of some noncommunicable, chronic diseases in the 21st century, between 1990 and 2020 the absolute number of deaths in the United States from noncommunicable disease will increase by 77 percent, from 28.1 million to 49.7 million.

An important shift in the burden of disease in the future is related to the huge impact of chronic disease around the world.[3] The World Health Organization (WHO) defines "burden of disease" as a combination of untimely death and disability.[4] The WHO Global Burden of Disease Study attempts to assess comprehensively current mortality and disabil-

Chapter 2: Demographic Trends and the Burden of Disease

Figure 2-9. Determinants of Health

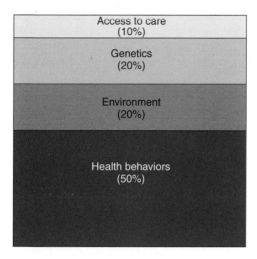

Source: IFTF; Centers for Disease Control and Prevention.

ity rates from diseases, injuries, and risk factors and to project them out to 2020. To assess the relative impact of different diseases, the study uses "1 year of healthy life lost" as a unit of measurement with which to compare disability and death from each disease. This approach reveals that the burden of a condition such as depression, alcohol dependence, or schizophrenia has been seriously underestimated by traditional approaches that take into account only deaths and not disabilities.

The overall effect of heart disease in terms of both death and disability rates will continue to be greater than that of any other illness. When looking only at mortality rates, cancer will continue to rank second. What is surprising in the current forecast is that—taking into account the extent to which an illness causes both death and disability—mental illness, especially unipolar major depression, will have a larger impact than cancer by the year 2010.

The burden of disease is also shifting from diseases caused by infectious organisms to disorders with behavioral causes, such as illnesses related to smoking and to alcohol abuse. It is estimated that lifestyle behaviors alone contribute to 50 percent of an individual's health status (see Figure 2-9). The biomedical model of health care, which focuses on a single causative agent for an illness and is concerned primarily with curing, is necessary but not sufficient. Much more needs to be done to create and implement effective health management and disease prevention programs. Our culture's current focus on wellness is encouraging but is primarily a phenomenon in the wealthier, more educated cohorts of society—which tend to have a better health status anyway.

ENDNOTES

[1] Adler, N. *Black Report*. Report of the Working Group on Inequalities in Health. London: DHSS, 1980.

[2] Wilkinson, R.G. Income distribution and life expectancy. *British Medical Journal* 1992; 304:165–68.

[3] *The Global Burden of Disease*. Murray, C.J.L, and Lopez, A.D. (eds.). Cambridge, MA: Harvard University Press, 1996.

[4] Unless otherwise noted, the information presented here is from unreleased United States Census data.

Chapter 2: Demographic Trends and the Burden of Disease

CHAPTER 3

Health Care's Demand Side

Will Future Growth Rates Be Like Those of the Past 5 Years or the Past 30?

The past 30 years in American health care have seen steady cost increases in excess of the growth of the rest of the economy: health care's share of GDP went from 5 percent in 1960 to nearly 14 percent in 1990, as shown in Figure 3-1. But after annual growth averaging more than 11 percent per year between 1960 and 1990 (3 percent above the nominal growth of the economy), annual growth in health care costs fell to 5.8 percent between 1992 and 1995 and has been falling each year since. For the first time in decades, health care costs appear to be stable as a share of GDP.[1] In the next 12 years, the key question is: Will the health sector grow at the rate of the past 5 years—just a little more than the economy—or will it resume the trend of the previous 30 years, when it grew much faster?

To understand the components of that cost growth, we need to know where the money comes from. The United States has had a balanced public-private health care financing system since the introduction of Medicaid and Medicare in 1965. Spending is fairly evenly split between government and the private sector, including out-of-pocket costs and insurance premiums paid by individuals. Any growth in overall health care costs will be a function of the growth in private costs, paid by both employers and individuals, and public costs.

THE PRIVATE SECTOR

So far it's the private sector that has experienced the greatest reversal in cost growth. From 1960 to 1990, private sector costs grew an average of 10.6 percent

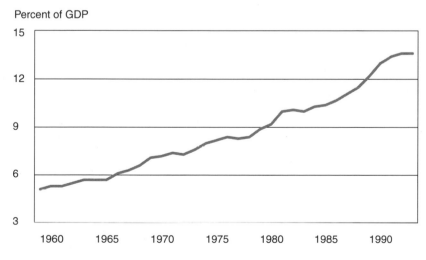

Figure 3-1. Total Health Care Expenditures as a Percentage of GDP, 1960–1965

Percent of GDP

Source: Health Care Financing Administration.

a year. From 1991 to 1995—in a period viewed by some as the triumph of market-based managed care and by others as the ultimate nadir of cost shifting from employers to consumers and government—private-sector health care costs fell below the growth rates of the rest of the economy, averaging under 5 percent per year[2] (see Figure 3-2). Many employers have seen an actual *decrease* in their health care expenditures. How was this achieved? First, employers passed more costs on to employees by demanding greater contributions in premiums and forcing higher copays and deductibles. Second, employers reduced the number of people for whom they provided insurance. But most of these cost decreases resulted from lower payments to health plans. In particular, HMOs and PPOs have actively intervened with care providers to lower costs and have become the staple form of insurance plan used by most employers, rather than the more traditional indemnity products.

THE PUBLIC SECTOR

From 1960 to 1990, public spending on health care grew at an annual average rate of 13.3 percent, about 3 percent more than in the private sector. But most of that difference related to the 1960s and 1970s when Medicare and Medicaid were expanding fast. In fact, the experience from 1991 to 1998 is in contrast to that in the early 1980s, when costs in the private sector grew faster than in the public sector. Recently the private sector has seen cost growth slow to below 5 percent, whereas the public sector has had average cost growths of over 9 percent for the past 5 years. The difference between the two has widened to nearly 5 percent, indicating that a greater share of health care spending is going to the public sector, and that public sector cost growth is of greater concern for the future.

While there are several reasons for this recent fast growth in public sector costs, a casual observer would notice that neither of the major public programs—Medicare and Medicaid—has been as quick to follow the private sector's lead in adopting HMOs or PPOs. Medicare's basic infrastructure supports an FFS cost-reimbursement system for virtually all types of services apart from hospital inpatient care, which was changed to a

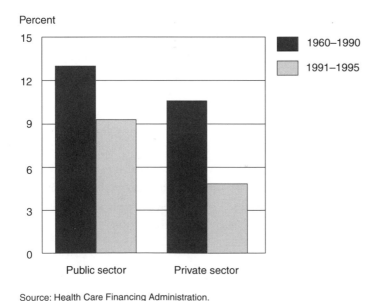

Figure 3-2. Average Annual Growth Rate of Health Care Costs by Sector

Percent

Legend:
- 1960–1990
- 1991–1995

Source: Health Care Financing Administration.

per-episode prospective payment system in 1983. This may partially explain why public program cost increases have not tailed off as they have in the private sector. Even if these are not the causative factors, they encapsulate two underlying legacies of Medicare and Medicaid—a typically FFS payment system and the peripherality of managed care—each of which will see dramatic changes over the next 12 years.

But the underlying question is whether the future will look more like the private sector's experience—health care cost growth in line with economic growth—or the public sector's experience of cost growth at 9 percent per year. The first possibility continues the recent 5-year trend. The second takes us back to the high cost-growth rates of the previous 30 years. Figure 3-3 shows

the share of GDP that would end up being consumed by health care under each scenario.

THE ISSUES: WHAT DRIVES FUTURE COST INCREASES?

Several factors are responsible for the slowing growth in health care costs in the early 1990s. They included the movement toward HMOs and PPOs, a reluctance to raise prices during the health care reform debate, and (arguably) a technological shift away from hospitalization. The question is whether these trends will continue.

In general we believe they will continue because the experiences and drives of consumers purchasing health care have changed since the mid-1990s. Some of these purchase factors include:

- *A more conservative Congress* passed a budget bill aimed in part at cutting back Medicare expenditures and delegating Medicaid decisions to the states. Managed care options will expand, quickly and involuntarily for people in Medicaid and more slowly for those in Medicare. Other entitlements such as Social Security are coming under consideration for future cuts in a political era when a balanced-budget mentality appears dominant.

- *Private (and some public sector) employers* have successfully maneuvered a majority of their workforce into HMO and PPO benefit products. They've also

Figure 3-3. Spending Under the 5-Year Trend or the 30-Year Trend (Health care expenditures as a share of GDP)

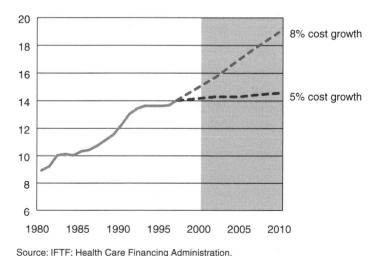

Source: IFTF; Health Care Financing Administration.

The Economy Is the Crucial Denominator

Because health expenditures react slowly to cost-cutting measures, the amount government and employers spend on health care goes up much faster than the rest of the economy in times of recession. This rise has a noticeable impact on both the share of GDP and the share of public sector revenues and private sector profits. Figure 3-4 shows that health care costs grew continually from 1981 to 1995, but the economy was less predictable. The difference in real health care spending growth and the growth in real GDP was greatest during recessions and least during economic booms. Historically, health care costs are regarded as a problem during and immediately after recessions while on average they increase only a little faster than economic growth.

Figure 3-4. Health Care Cost Increases Get Noticed During Recessions (Real changes in national health expenditure [NHE] as compared to real changes in GDP over time)

Percent

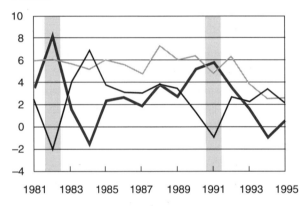

— Change in GDP, in constant 1992 dollars
— Real change in NHE
— Difference between NHE and GDP

Source: Health Care Financing Administration, U.S. Bureau of Labor.

either prodded health plans (intermediaries) into more aggressive cost-containment efforts with providers or have increasingly purchased coverage from plans that have taken that stance. Now that employers know they can influence costs, they are not likely to loosen that control.

■ *Consumers* experienced a steady decrease in their share of national health care spending from 1960 to 1990, even though health care costs increased as a share of household spending. But with a combination of fewer employers offering insurance and, of those who do, more demanding premium contributions and increased deductibles and copays, consumers are picking up more of the financial slack. They are likely to be more cost conscious in the future.

■ *Providers are more "sophisticated."* While higher health care costs ultimately translate into higher provider incomes, in the past 5 years payers have clearly communicated their demands for cost containment. In this equation, specific providers may be rewarded for reducing costs—despite the myriad pressures to increase costs—and all providers are aware of that pressure.

Although these factors indicate that a slowing of the underlying growth in health care costs has taken place, several traditional factors ensure that cost inflation will not die easily. For instance:

■ The vast majority of providers are paid on some type of an *FFS basis*. FFS medicine stimulates increased use of services in contrast to capitation, the most extreme form of managed care payment. Although pure FFS medicine is in decline, most forms of provider payment still encourage more utilization of services rather than less.

■ New, and usually more expensive, *drugs and medical technologies* are becoming available all the time. Use of these drugs and technologies tends to spread quickly whether or not they are cost-effective.

■ A *growing labor force*, as evidenced by the number of both high-cost employees (e.g., physicians) and low-cost employees in the health care industry, increased at an average annual rate of 3.78 percent between 1980 and 1998. That's 2.73 percent more than the rate

of population growth, yet overall wage rates have remained roughly constant. So as more resources go to health care employment, it appears that the supply-driven demand demonstrated during the 1970s is still in evidence.[3]

THE FORECAST: REAL COST GROWTH AT 1 PERCENT

There are good reasons to believe that the dramatic growth rate of the past 30 years has come to an end. But there are still sufficient factors to warrant suspicion that the experience of the private sector—a reduction in health cost rates below overall economic growth—over the past 5 years is unlikely to be replicated across the system.

Overall, we forecast that health care expenditures during the next 12 years are likely to grow at 6.4 percent annually—equivalent to just under 1 percent more than nominal GDP growth. If this prediction is correct, then health care, which currently consumes 14 percent of GDP, will reach 15.25 percent in 10 years and just over 15.6 percent in 2010 (see Figure 3-5). Within that steady growth, the gap between rates of cost growth in the private and public sectors will narrow.

Why will the gap narrow? So far, much of the private sector's gains have come at the expense of consumers, the public sector, and providers. For instance, there are relatively fewer people insured by their own or their family's employers now

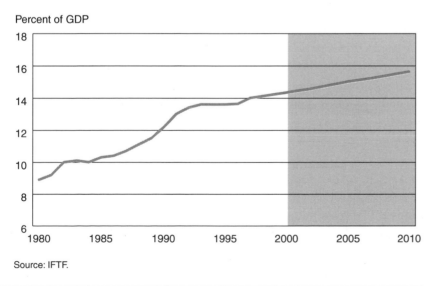

Figure 3-5. Projection of Future Health Care Spending
(Health care expenditures as a share of GDP)

Percent of GDP

Source: IFTF.

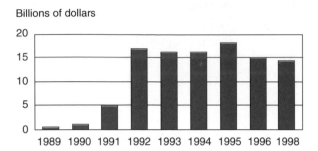

Figure 3-6. DSH Spending Explodes in the Early 1990s

Billions of dollars

Source: U.S. General Accounting Office, The Urban Institute.

Figure 3-7 shows that the cost reductions have resulted in disproportionately higher benefits to private payers at the expense of public payers.

We don't believe that this discrepancy between cost growth in the public and private sectors can continue at the 5 percent differential seen in the 1990s. It looks like the gains made in the private sector at the public sector's expense were mostly a one-time gain, and the gap is now starting to narrow.

Evidence of such a reversal is accumulating. Private insurance premiums increased between 3 percent and 8 percent in 1998, due mostly to poor margins among health plans and to increased utilization of pharmaceuticals and physician services. Meanwhile, the Medicare and Medicaid cost increases in excess of 10 percent seen during the early 1990s slowed to 8 percent and less than 5 percent, respectively, in 1996 and 1997. The 1997 balanced-budget legislation attempt to put an overall cap on the growth of Medicare costs at 6 percent for the period from 1998 to 2002 should cause a further reduction in overall cost increases in the public sector. This reduction in Medicare spending should put more pressure on providers, who in turn will try to transfer their costs to the private sector.

We forecast that private sector cost growth will move closer to the 3 to 6 percent range over the next 7 to 12 years, and public sector cost increases will end up in the 6 to 9 percent range. Hence, our forecast of overall costs averages 6.4 percent per year.

than there were 10 years ago. The increase in the number of working uninsured and the fact that most employers are demanding greater contributions toward insurance costs mean that more pressure is put on safety-net providers, such as public hospitals and inner-city academic medical centers (AMCs). Consequently, the financial health of these institutions has suffered and the amount of compensation the government has paid out in disproportionate share payments (DSH) made to hospitals that deliver a higher than average amount of uncompensated care reflects this impact (see Figure 3-6). Similarly, the Medicaid expansion of the late 1980s added about 10 million people to the program at a time when fewer people were receiving coverage from employers.

In addition, the mainstream Medicare and Medicaid programs have either experienced cost shifting from private insurers or simply haven't shared as greatly in the productivity improvements that providers, especially hospitals, have experienced over the past few years.

Chapter 3: Health Care's Demand Side

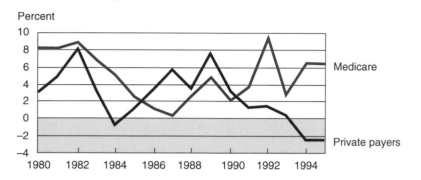

Figure 3-7. Medicare Gets a Worse Deal in the 1990s
(Average annual per capita growth in Medicare and private health insurance spending in hospitals)

Source: Health Care Financing Administration.

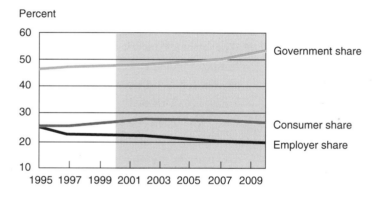

Figure 3-8. Share of Costs Borne by Government, Employers, and Consumers

Source: IFTF; Health Care Financing Administration.

Why will costs stay at that level rather than go much higher or even back to the 30-year trend? In the private sector, employers and other payers now understand that they don't simply have to accept large cost increases year after year. Meanwhile, recent Medicare legislation appears to be the most comprehensive attempt yet to implement cost containment across the entire program. Previous

efforts simply squeezed one part of the Medicare cost balloon and let it bulge out elsewhere.[4]

Nonetheless, given the greater pressures on the Medicare and Medicaid programs and the traditional ability of providers to take advantage of the comparative inflexibility of these programs, we project that—although cost growth will slow—the government's share of all health care expenditures will increase rapidly. The government's share of spending on health, *excluding* the government as employer, will increase from around 46.75 percent today to as much as 47.5 percent in 2002, when the current Medicare budget plan expires, and to as much as 52 percent by 2010.[5]

Consumers will be the other major source of increased spending because they will be paying more for health care. Currently, out-of-pocket costs (direct spending on medical services) are $182 billion a year, or about 18 percent of total health care expenditures. In addition, individuals pay $62.5 billion in private insurance premiums, either for their primary insurance, as a contribution to what their employer provides, or for Medigap coverage.[6] Combined, these costs account for 25 percent of total health care spending.

Because of the reduction in scope of benefits, increased consumer demand for over-the-counter (OTC) medical products and complementary services such as chiropractic care, and the slightly higher growth rate of individual health insurance versus group insurance, we forecast that this share of total spending will rise to as much as 28 percent by 2002. After that, growth in the public sector will absorb some of the increase and it will fall back to 26.5 percent by 2010. But for the next 5 years, health care will rise as a share of overall consumer spending.

Ten years from today, employers will be paying a smaller share of overall costs and government and consumers will be paying a greater proportion (see Figure 3-8).

THE SIGNIFICANCE OF OUR COST FORECAST FOR THE REST OF OUR 10-YEAR OUTLOOK

We broadly agree with forecasts suggesting that the health care cost problem is not going to go away. The nominal rate of health care cost growth for the period 1992 to 2010 will be about 6.4 percent, or 1 percent over GDP, as opposed to 3 percent over GDP for the period 1960 to 1990. But we believe (with some temerity) this relatively slower cost growth may not be the dominant issue for the next 10 years. The period up to 2010 is likely to be a cost-containment hiatus given the impact of the soon-to-retire baby boomers in the years between 2010 and 2030.

WILD CARDS

- Risk selection sinks Medicare savings: Medicare managed care ends up with medical savings accounts (MSAs), PSNs, and HMOs cream-skimming on a noticeable scale.

- Cost-reduction strategies in fast-growing parts of Medicare such as SNFs or

home health and outpatient services either don't work or are counterproductive because they create fast-growing exceptions. Those rapidly growing programs are joined by other new programs like telemedicine, which are equally expensive.

- Cost shifting to providers and public payers causes a collapse of the safety net, forcing large influxes of federal funding to several inner-city areas.

- The next recession is deeper than anticipated, requiring more services for the indigent and hence a greater share of government revenue and GDP for health care while taxes and other revenues decline.

- The weapons are taken out of the hands of managed care. A combination of legal and regulatory restrictions on health plans, such as "any-willing-provider" laws, and bans on capitation and utilization review tilt negotiating power back toward providers.

- A provider surplus, plus aggressive HMOs, plus Medicare's actually sticking to 6 percent cost increases and Medicaid's getting tougher, keep costs below our forecast and below 4.5 percent. As a consequence, health care shrinks as a share of GDP.

- The technology revolution increases the rate of economic growth. Health care costs shrink as a share of GDP because GDP grows so quickly.

ENDNOTES

[1] Since the mid-1980s, the economy has generally grown at an annual rate of 5.5 percent in nominal terms (2.5 percent real growth and 3 percent inflation). Thus, for health costs to maintain their share of GDP they would have to grow at an average annual rate of 5.5 percent in nominal terms.

[2] That is, less than 5.5 percent, the average growth of the economy in nominal terms (not adjusted for inflation).

[3] Fuchs, V. R., and Kramer, M. J. Determinants of expenditure for physicians services. In Fuchs, V. R. *The Health Economy.* Cambridge, MA: Harvard University Press, 1986.

[4] Medicaid too appears to be growing more slowly. However, the recent falls in Medicaid cost growth (i.e., to below 4 percent in 1996) have come during an economic expansion. Because Medicaid costs grow fastest during recessions, we forecast Medicaid growth to remain at about 8 percent.

[5] This does not include the government's spending as an employer. We consider that spending as private health insurance (as does the Health Care Financing Administration [HCFA] in some versions of the national health expenditure [NHE]) and believe that it will increase at the rate of private spending. In 1995, government spending on insurance for federal, state, and local government employees amounted to roughly $58 billion of the $242 billion spent by employers on private health insurance in 1995. If this were to be counted as part of government health expenditures, it would mean that the government accounted for 52 percent of health expenditures in 1995.

[6] This does not include $16 billion paid as premiums by individuals for Part B of Medicare, which is included in our Medicare numbers.

CHAPTER 4

Health Insurance

The Three-Tiered Model

The American health insurance system developed out of a need for hospitals and physicians to make their product affordable to ordinary people. Health insurance first became a reality for Americans in the 1930s with the creation of specialized health insurance companies—the Blue Cross and Blue Shield plans. The system was given a boost when health insurance became an employment benefit during and after World War II, and when Medicare (for the elderly) and Medicaid (for the poor) were created in 1965. It was this indemnity-based system of mixed public and private insurance sources that constituted the mainstream of American health care until the early 1980s. Only in some regions, notably in the West, were any substantial number of people enrolled in the prepaid health plans that were later called HMOs.

During the 1970s and 1980s, a series of legislative and court decisions fostered the growth of selective contracting. Selective contracting allowed insurance plans, which came to be known as PPOs and HMOs, to contract with networks of providers. The plans could arrange the contracts at a predetermined price and reimburse providers for their services in a number of different ways, still including (but not limited to) a traditional FFS model. Generally, the Medicare and Medicaid programs were not included in these arrangements.

By the early 1990s, the cost advantages that HMOs and PPOs afforded employers were great enough that most large employers, such as the California Public Employees Retirement System (CalPERS), moved their employees to this type of insurance arrangement. This caused a rapid growth in the numbers of people enrolled in HMOs and PPOs, and later in hybrid models like point-of-service (POS) programs. By 1995, most companies had moved their workers away from indemnity plans, and by 1998 more than 70 million people were enrolled in HMO plans (see Figures 4-1 and 4-2).

Moving employees into managed care plans was not employers' only response to rising health care costs. They also offered insurance to fewer employees. The proportion of nonelderly who had employment-based insurance fell from 69.2 percent in 1987 to 63.5 percent in 1993 (see Figure 4-3).[1] Insurance coverage has stayed at this level despite the large number of new jobs created during the economic expansion from 1992 to 1997. This erosion of health insurance as an employee benefit has been particularly severe for employees with no more than a high school education (see Figure 4-4).

*Figure 4-1. HMO Membership Takes Off in the 1990s
(Number of HMO enrollees in millions)*

Source: Group Health Administration of America, Interstudy, American Association of Health Plans.

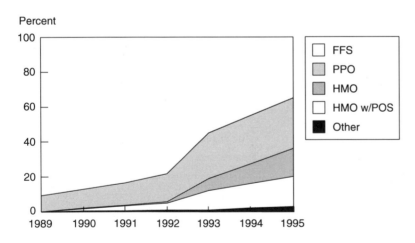

Figure 4-2. Type of Plan That Covered Most Employees of Companies with 100+ Workers

Source: IFTF Employer Surveys, 1989, 1992, 1993, 1995.

What has also changed over the past few years is the number of people who are uninsured. This number, which typically increases during recessions and decreases during economic expansions, appears to be increasing during expansions. This increase suggests that, in the current expansion, any income effects (people buying insurance as a result of higher incomes or employers offering health insurance benefits as a result of a tighter labor marker) or price effects (people buying more health insurance when it becomes relatively cheaper) are being outweighed by:

- structural shifts away from employer-sponsored insurance, such as more part-time workers and more workers in smaller firms (see Figure 4-5).

- the sharp decline in health insurance provided by small businesses (see Figure 4-6), which already offered less health insurance than larger firms (see Figure 4-7). This decline occurred in part because many jobs in small businesses are now in the service sector, where employers offer fewer benefits than in the manufacturing sector.

- the underlying price effect: employers and individuals drop insurance coverage because of increasing costs relative to real wages, which are still below their 1989 level.

So the plight of the uninsured, which has been a focus of health policy throughout the century and led to the creation of Medicare and Medicaid, will remain unresolved if current trends persist. The numbers of uninsured have

Figure 4-3. Employment-Based Insurance Is Falling . . .
(Percentage of nonelderly adults with employer-sponsored health insurance)

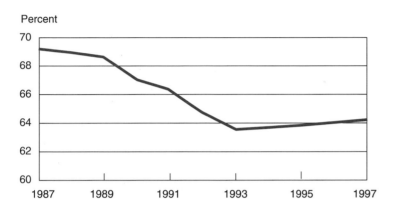

Source: Little, J. S. *New England Economic Review*, 1995.

*Figure 4-4. . . . and It's the Least Educated Who've Borne the Brunt
of the Decline (Percentage of full-time, male workers with health benefits, by
educational attainment)*

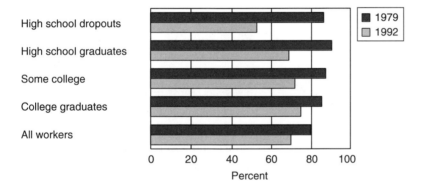

Source: Little, J. S. *New England Economic Review*, 1995.

been growing fairly steadily, reaching 44 million people in 1998. This figure correlates to approximately 15 percent of the population's being uninsured at any one time, and 7 to 9 percent being uninsured for a year or more. Although there is some dispute over the calculation,[2] it appears that the number of uninsured has recently been rising by about 750,000 per year, a growth rate of 2 percent as compared to an overall population growth of 1 percent. However, the absolute number of uninsured increased about 2 million each year during the 1990–1992 recession.

THE ISSUES: HOW WILL PEOPLE RECEIVE HEALTH INSURANCE?

Both the source of health insurance funding and the type of insurance coverage people receive have great influence on the health care system. Some of the factors determining how people receive health insurance over the next 12 years are predictable. These include the source of funding: employee-funded health insurance will remain the mainstream, and most people will have their insurance paid for by the same source it comes from now.

An assessment of the sources of health insurance for Americans (see Figure 4-8) shows that in 1998 approximately 168 million Americans (62 percent) received private health insurance from their employer or purchased it themselves. Of the remainder, 28 million (10 percent) were in the Medicaid program, 38 million (14 percent) were in Medicare, and about 44 million (16 percent) had no

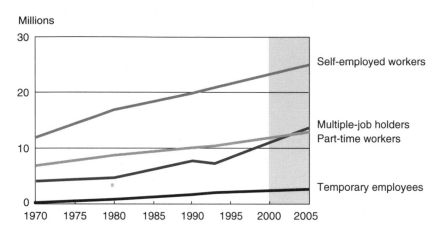

Figure 4-5. *The Flexible Workforce Is Growing Quickly*

Millions

Self-employed workers

Multiple-job holders
Part-time workers

Temporary employees

Source: IFTF; U.S. Bureau of Labor Statistics, Employment and Earnings.

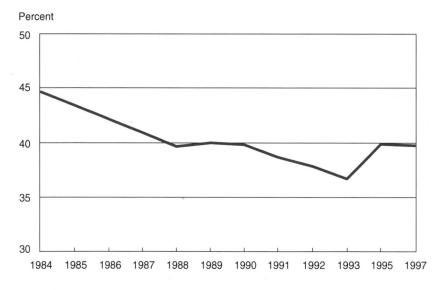

Figure 4-6. *Small Business Drops Health Benefits*
(Percentage of employees at firms of <100 receiving health benefits from their employer over time)

Percent

Source: Employee Benefits Research Institute, Small Business Administration.

health insurance and relied on self-pay, county and local programs, or charity. [3]

Sources of insurance will remain fairly stable. For the next 5 years, we know who the Medicare population will be; any future policy changes related to eligibility will not kick in until late in the next decade. In the near future, employment-based insurance will remain the predominant form of insurance for most people under 65. There will be a continuing group of Medicaid recipients and uninsured, but their numbers cannot be known for certain. The major categories of Medicare, Medicaid, uninsured, and private health insurance will remain the core sources of coverage, or lack thereof.

However, the question is not only from which source do people receive health insurance—we must also ask what form does that insurance take? During the past few years, most people with employer-based insurance have moved from indemnity plans into a variety of more complex models, including several types of open-panel HMOs and PPOs. The shift from indemnity to PPO and HMO models will continue, with the shift accelerating in the public programs.

Contrary to popular opinion, the growth in PPOs and HMOs was not primarily due to an increase in the number of enrollees of traditional staff- and group-model health plans, such as Kaiser Permanente or Harvard Pilgrim Health Plan. Instead, most of the growth came from independent practice association–based (IPA) HMOs that developed new contracting arrangements with community providers (see Figure 4-9). In other words,

*Figure 4-7. Few Small Business Employees Find Insurance at Work . . . or Anywhere Else
(Source of insurance coverage by size of employer, 1997)*

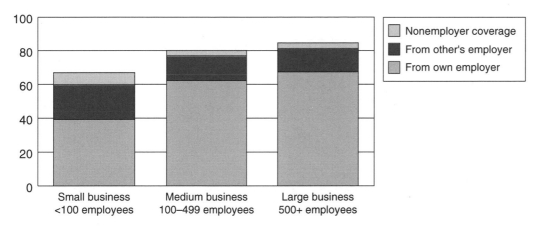

Source: Employee Benefits Research Institute Issue Brief, December 1998.

Figure 4-8. Sources of Health Insurance for Americans over Time

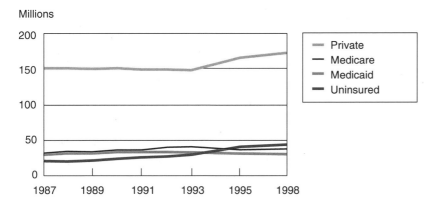

Source: IFTF, using data from Health Care Financing Administration, Employee Benefits Research
Institute, and Current Population Survey.

the delivery system used by the new
intermediaries was the same one that Blue
Cross, Blue Shield, and traditional indemnity systems had been using all along.

In the mid-1990s, more Medicare and
Medicaid recipients enrolled in HMOs.
Some state governments forced Medicaid
recipients to join HMOs, and it became
more attractive for private-sector health

plans to recruit senior citizens into specialized HMOs. This "Medicare risk contracting" was increasingly profitable for
commercial health plans, particularly in
areas where Medicare's average costs were
high. For each member enrolled, HMOs
were paid 95 percent of the average costs
of a Medicare recipient in that particular
county—a reimbursement policy that
encouraged the recruitment of seniors in
high-cost markets such as Los Angeles,
Miami, and New York City. Membership
of Medicare recipients in risk-contracting
HMOs grew from 4 percent at the end of
1989 to 6 percent at the end of 1994, to
13 percent at the beginning of 1998 (see
Figure 4-10). Medicare recipients are
now allowed to join other types of health
plans, such as PPOs, under the new
Medicare+Choice program.

Two major issues, then, have influenced
our forecast for health insurance. One is
the *source* of insurance. The major sources

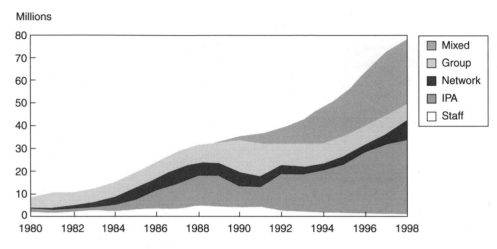

Figure 4-9. It's Been the IPAs That Have Grown Fastest
(HMO enrollment growth split by IPA and network models versus group and staff models)

Millions

Legend:
- Mixed
- Group
- Network
- IPA
- Staff

Source: IFTF, using data from Interstudy.

Figure 4-10. Enrollment Growth in Medicare Risk (TEFRA) HMOs

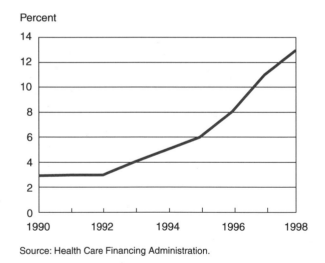

Percent

Source: Health Care Financing Administration.

ucts—indemnity, PPO, and HMO—the distinction among different types of HMOs, PPOs, POSs, and all the rest of the players in the alphabet soup is becoming irrelevant. Continued innovation in the benefit plans' contractual arrangements will rapidly erode the distinction among the classic gatekeeper HMOs, PPOs, POSs, and other models of managed care.

THE FORECAST: SOURCE OF INSURANCE —WHERE ARE THE PEOPLE? . . .

PRIVATE INSURANCE

The downward trend in the number of people with employment-based insurance and the upward trend in the numbers with Medicaid and those who are uninsured will remain constant over the next

of health insurance will remain fairly constant through 2010, although the relative proportions will change slightly.

The other is the *type* of insurance. Although we estimate the numbers enrolled in the classically defined prod-

What's Behind Medicaid's Growth?

The Medicaid program has grown in both size and complexity since its inception in 1965.[4] The program now accounts for about 15 percent of all health care spending ($188 billion in 1999) and covers 36 million people, primarily with four major types of coverage:

1. acute medical insurance coverage

2. coverage for the disabled, including residential care for the long-term mentally disabled

3. long-term care for the poor elderly (those who have "spent down" to poverty level and need nursing home care)

4. state Medicaid programs paying the Medicare Part B insurance premiums for poor elderly and disabled (known as dual eligibles)

Sixty-five percent of people enrolled in Medicaid are in the first category, and 65 percent of the money is spent on the 35 percent in the last three categories. As that spending tends to fall outside of the traditional acute care model, it is difficult to include in managed care programs.

A series of legislated eligibility expansions in the late 1980s, followed by the 1990–1992 recession, increased the number of people covered by Medicaid from 23 million in 1987 to 36 million in 1996. Currently, about 28 million people use Medicaid as their primary source of health insurance (our model counts the dual eligibles in the Medicare numbers). Federal legislation in 1996 gave states far more freedom to alter Medicaid plans, both in terms of implementing new benefit arrangements and in changing eligibility levels. Meanwhile several states, notably Tennessee, had already moved their Medicaid population into managed care programs.[5] Most other states have announced an intention to do the same, and we forecast that about 60 percent of Medicaid recipients will be in managed care plans by 2005, although they will account for only 35 percent of spending.

The 1997 Balanced Budget Act also gave the states funding to increase the number of children covered by health insurance. States may use these funds to increase Medicaid eligibility levels for children or they may create separate child health programs.

10 years. The number receiving health insurance from employers will decrease, *as a proportion of the overall population,* at 1 percent every 5 years, from about 59 percent in 1997 to about 56 percent in 2010 (see Figure 4-11). Due to overall population growth, their total number will increase by about 13 million.

MEDICARE

Meanwhile, the population insured through Medicare will increase at a slightly faster rate than the rate of overall population growth, increasing from just under 38 million (14.2 percent of the population) currently to 45 million in 2007 (15.5 percent) and 49 million in 2010 (16.8 percent). While the numbers of the elderly will increase, the fastest-growing segment of the Medicare population is now the disabled, which is growing at 6 percent annually. Considering that no eligibility changes were made in 1997, a policy that is unlikely to change during the next several years, we think that Medicare will continue to cover people over 65 years of age, at least until 2010. There are now 34 million Americans over 65 and there will be 40 million in 2010. The significant growth in the population over 65 years old, owing to the baby boom after World War II, will not begin until 2010 and will continue until 2040.

MEDICAID

There are now about 28 million Americans (10.3 percent of the population) who use Medicaid as their primary source of health insurance. That number does not include the nearly 6 million people who are eligible for both Medicaid and Medicare. It also does not include an estimated 6 million additional people who are eligible for the Medicaid program but are not enrolled in it—we classify these people among the uninsured. The rate of growth of the Medicaid population depends on both federal and state government policies and the economy, and it is notoriously

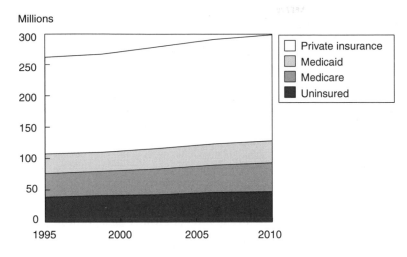

Figure 4-11. Future Sources of Health Insurance for Americans

Millions

Legend:
- Private insurance
- Medicaid
- Medicare
- Uninsured

Source: IFTF, based on data and projections from Health Care Financing Administration, Urban Institute, Lewin Inc., and Congressional Budget Office.

difficult to forecast. However, we do not forecast a substantial expansion in Medicaid eligibility other than for some children covered under the 1997 Balanced Budget Act.

We estimate that the number served by Medicaid will grow from 28 million to 34 million by 2010.[6] Several factors could inflate this forecast, including a faster uptake of children into Medicaid or a severe recession that would cause an expansion in the ranks of the poor. However, states now freed from federal mandates could tighten eligibility requirements, which would reduce the number of people served.

THE UNINSURED

The uninsured will still constitute a sizable proportion of Americans, but our core forecast is that they will continue to be about 15 percent of the population.

Although counting the number of uninsured is problematic, their number appears to be increasing at about 750,000 people per year. Because health insurance costs have dropped in the past 3 years, we project that this number will fall over the next 5 years, although a likely recession may keep the average growth at 750,000.

There will also be a modest impact on Medicaid as between 1.5 and 2 million children receive coverage over the next 5 years through the Children's Health Insurance Program (CHIP) provision of the 1997 Balanced Budget Act (10 million of the 42 million currently uninsured are under 18 years of age).

We forecast that by 2002 the numbers of uninsured will increase from the current 43 million to around 44 million. After 2002, the average rate of increase will decline, partly because of the shifting age structure in the population. Lack of insurance is most common among people of age 18 to 34 years, and most of the baby boomers will be age 40 to 60 years by the next decade. Overall, we estimate that the rate of growth in the uninsured will be close to an additional 500,000 per year through 2010. We estimate that, in 2007, 16 percent of Americans (46.4 million) will be uninsured, a percentage that will rise to 16.1 percent or 47.9 million in 2010.

The important factor in these projections is the *proportion* of the population that is uninsured at any one time. About 21 million of the 42 million uninsured will be uninsured for a year or more. Twice that number will be uninsured at some time over a 2-year period.

. . . AND WHAT TYPE OF INSURANCE WILL THEY HAVE?

Figure 4-12. The Future Is Much More of the Present
(Type of insurance coverage for the insured)

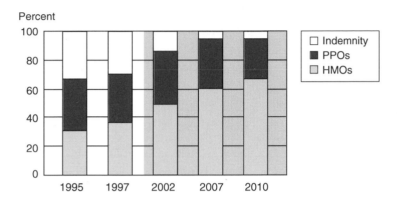

Source: IFTF.

Figure 4-13. HMO Descendants Move from Mainstream to Majority
(Number of Americans in HMOs, by source of insurance)

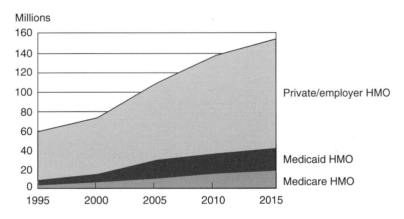

Source: IFTF.

While the distinctions among indemnity, PPO, and HMO are breaking down, the number of people moving toward managed care have been counted in the increase in HMO membership, and that's how managed care enrollment will be forecast in the near future. Figure 4-12 shows the change in type of insurance coverage held by the insured over the next decade.

Among people with private insurance HMO membership has been growing at about 7 percent each year during the 1990s. We expect that rate to remain constant until 2002, then drop to 5 percent from 2002 to 2007, and to 4 percent after 2007. Indemnity programs increasingly will turn into PPOs, and PPO membership will increase to about 60 million by 2002. But by 2010 the number will decline to below 50 million as PPO members begin to move into HMOs. However, the distinctions among these products will be hard to discern by then and we will call them "HMO descendants."

Medicare and Medicaid HMO enrollment is likely to grow considerably faster (see Figure 4-13). We estimate that enrollment in Medicare risk HMOs will continue to grow at a consistent rate of about 90,000 insured lives a month. That trend will result in about 25 percent of seniors being in Medicare risk HMOs by 2002—doubling the current percentage—and about 33 percent by 2007.[7] The variety of managed care plans offered by the private sector to these seniors will increase to include

POSs and even PPOs. Most of the rest of the Medicare population will remain in an FFS program, but a small minority may choose alternatives, such as MSAs or private indemnity plans. Medicaid HMO enrollment will increase much faster, as the recipients will be given no choice and will not need to be sold memberships one by one. We project that virtually all the nondisabled adults and children in Medicaid will be moved into HMOs by 2002. This process has already started, and despite some false starts, within 5 years it should be nearly complete, with as many as 63 percent of Medicaid recipients in HMOs.[8]

Overall, we forecast that HMOs will cement their position as the dominant form of health insurance product over the next decade. PPOs will have some durability as an indemnity-like insurance product, particularly within the upper echelons of the employee population. Pure indemnity will decline rapidly in importance, remaining viable only in the Medicare program and for a tiny percentage of the employed.

But the real importance behind these distinctions in health insurance models will fade by the early years of the next century. Two key issues will be of concern to insurers in 2010:

- What the components of the benefits package will be, in terms of the insured's obligations such as coinsurance, deductibles, and copayments.

- The way in which insurance plans pay the providers.

The first issue, benefits packages and the insured's obligations, will reflect the underlying tiering that is developing among consumers in the population as a whole (see Chapter 9). We look at the second question, provider reimbursement, in Chapter 5.

TIERING WILL INCREASE

Three types of insurance models (see Figure 4-14) are likely to develop based on the employment status and wealth of the participants:

- *Carriage trade indemnity or PPO, including traditional Medicare:* These will remain traditional programs with high deductibles and coinsurance, copayments, and free choice of providers.

- *HMO descendants:* Most Americans will have excellent benefits in terms of low or no deductibles, and low copayments (the current HMO standard) if they stay within the provider network and work through their plans' referral processes (be it through a gatekeeper physician or a nurse). The option to self-refer to other providers will be covered in general, but at a lower percentage of reimbursement with higher copayments and most likely higher coinsurance.

- *The low tier:* This tier will include most Medicaid enrollees, who face a more restrictive set of provider choices but with better access to them than they've experienced in the traditional program. The providers for this group will be dealing with most of the uninsured. There will also be continued

Figure 4-14. Tiers 'R' Us . . . and Will Be

Source: IFTF.

ment Models: Between Finance and Delivery" section in Chapter 5.

WILD CARDS

- A severe, protracted recession increases the number of uninsured and Medicaid eligibles by 75 percent each.

- Universal health insurance legislation is enacted, reducing the number of uninsured to nearly zero.

- Health insurance premiums become a taxable benefit; employers stop providing coverage and abandon the market as purchasers.

- MSAs, vouchers for Medicare, and other individual-based buying become significant forces, changing the group nature of the insurance market.

- HMO enrollment growth in either Medicare or the commercial market slows substantially or even declines due to legislative, market, or other pressures.

- A national health insurance system is adopted; private-sector insurance is eliminated.

but limited efforts to help uninsured individuals and small groups buy into these low-tier plans.

To see how these factors will translate into reimbursement and affect the provider system, see the "Reimburse

ENDNOTES

[1] Employee Benefits Research Institute (EBRI) analysis of 1987–96 Current Population Survey (CPS).

[2] For example, the two main surveys used to calculate this number, the CPS and the National Health Insurance Survey (NHIS), count uninsured children in different ways. They also count veterans, who potentially could use Veterans Affairs hospitals, differently. In another example of the mystique around this number, the survey questionnaire was changed in the 1995 CPS, which led to its showing an apparently large rise in the number of people receiving coverage at work while many other surveys were revealing the opposite.

[3] About 20 million (7 percent) buy health insurance themselves.

[4] The expansion in Medicaid eligibility in the late 1980s, which increased the population covered from about 19 million to closer to 30 million, kept the number of uninsured lower than it would otherwise have been. Few of those new Medicaid recipients had previously been uninsured—in fact most of them had been insured by an employer—but this expansion of Medicaid eligibility did make a one-time impact on the underlying trend of uninsurance.

[5] Until the 1996 legislation, it was necessary for states to receive a waiver from the federal government to make substantial changes in their Medicaid programs. Several waivers were granted, including one that allowed Tennessee to introduce the TennCare managed care program for Medicaid recipients and the uninsured.

[6] There is some controversy over forecasting Medicaid enrollment. The Congressional Budget Office (CBO) estimates annual Medicaid growth of 2.7 percent. The Urban Institute reworked the CBO number in 1997 and established, to our satisfaction, that CBO had overestimated the growth in the core Medicaid populations of Aid to Families with Dependent Children (AFDC) mothers and children and disabled people. They projected a 1.6 percent annual growth rate, which we've used here.

[7] This is much lower than several other estimates, including the CBO's estimate. But it is revised up from our 1995 projection, which had Medicare HMO growth stalling at around 25 percent. The upward revision takes into account future changes in adjusted average per capita cost (AAPCC) rates, the abolition of the 50/50 rule, the boost to rural AAPCC rates, and the PSN legislation that will make it easier to set up the infrastructure to enroll seniors in smaller markets. One major brake on Medicare Risk enrollment is the likely institution of risk adjustment for government-paid premiums after 2000. This could make enrolling healthy seniors a good deal less profitable than it is now. In any event, HMO penetration will not approach that seen in the employer market.

[8] This includes prepaid health plans and HMOs but not primary care case management, which we regard as an addendum to the regular FFS program.

CHAPTER 5

Health Care Providers
Themes of the Future Delivery System

The mixture of physicians, hospitals, and other providers that makes up the American health care delivery system has never been a well-organized entity. We are a few years into what we perceive will be 15 to 20 years of profound change in the way health care providers are organized. This period of change will occupy all of our forecast period up to 2010, and the outcome of those changes will be of profound importance for the future well beyond 2010. Although patients will be involved in all stages, both as active agents and as passive recipients of change, most of the action will be driven externally by employers, governments, and health insurers, with various players in the system trying to create organizations that will survive and even prosper in the future. Several key backdrops frame this system:

■ *Continued organizational change.* A combination of the demands of employers, the rise of managed care, the recommendations of consultants, and the infusion of Wall Street capital into the health care system has led to a desire for new models of health care delivery. Current providers are trying to make sure that they will be in the game for the long term. Consequently, there has been a rash of mergers, acquisi-

tions, and new initiatives among all sectors of the market. This activity has been as prevalent among nonprofit organizations as it has been among their Wall Street–funded brethren. It presages a slow transition from a world of independent entities to one of more corporate systems. Between here and there have been—and will be—many false starts, poor investment decisions, and organizational disasters.

■ *The role of intermediaries.* Health care plans, disease management companies, case managers, and other management organizations will become much more important in directing patients to providers and in intervening and directing the activities of care providers and patients. There is a possibility that providers will attempt to circumvent the intermediaries and go directly to such end payers as employers or Medicare. There is also a possibility that, as patients become more engaged in their care, they will influence the behavior of these intermediaries as well as that of their providers.

■ *An oversupply of hospital beds and a surplus of physicians.* America has far more hospital beds than it uses, and many more than it needs. Whether or not this situation is a surplus to some normative "need," the overall market effect is that providers increasingly will be working in a buyer's market rather than the seller's market that has existed for the past 6 decades.

■ *Control over medical management* will be the main arena of interorganizational conflict in the medium-term future. Physicians and providers have lost substantial organizational, financial, and clinical control to health plans and payers, but they have been building systems to win back some of that control. Control over medical management will be the central arena in which this power struggle plays out. The shift in locus of decision making away from individual clinicians to other entities will continue. The question is how far and how fast will that shift go, and exactly who will direct medical decision making.

Assuming these four major themes—overcapacity in the system, continued change among all organizations, the evolving role of the intermediary, and a battle over control of medical management—this chapter forecasts the future roles of intermediaries, the new models of payment to providers and care organizations, and the structure of service-delivery organizations.

INTERMEDIARIES

BACKGROUND: THE CONVERGENCE OF OPEN NETWORKS AND THE DEMISE OF VERTICAL INTEGRATION

The past 15 years have produced a dramatic change in the commercial insurance market and we are now seeing the beginning of a similar change in the Medicare and Medicaid systems. HMOs, PPOs, and POS plans, which limit patients' access to physicians and services through financial incentives and gatekeepers, have become the dominant form of health insurance for employees and their families. Similarly restrictive plans have been able to increase enrollment in Medicaid and even in Medicare. However, most enrollment growth has not been in the classic prepaid health plans—the staff- and group-model HMOs—but rather in IPA-based HMOs that use mainstream community physicians and hospitals.

This pattern surprised many observers who thought that the cohesiveness and internal controls of group and staff plans would give them a competitive advantage over the IPA models. However, IPA models have succeeded in controlling provider costs, meaning that there has been little competitive advantage of the staff-model HMOs. Providing access to the same providers that patients were already seeing has been the IPA models' biggest advantage in selling their products. The shift toward IPA-based HMOs has significantly changed what most pundits thought the managed care landscape was going to look like (see Figure 5-1).

Figure 5-1. Managed Competition: How It Was Supposed to Be

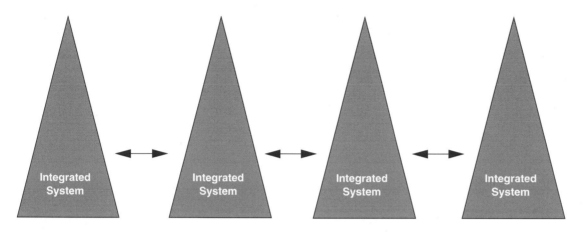

World of:
- competition between vertically integrated systems
- exclusive relationships
- empowered consumers

How It Really Is

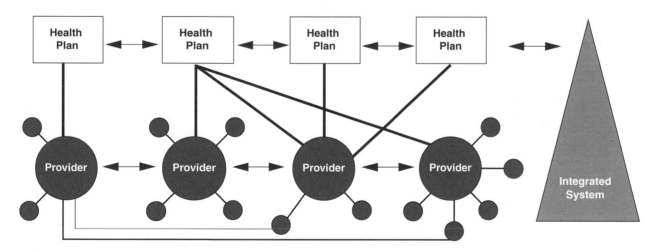

World of:
- horizontally integrated delivery systems
- nonexclusive relationships
- competition among plans and providers
- confused consumers

Source: IFTF.

Virtually all HMOs—with the notable exception of Kaiser Permanente and the few other group- and staff-model HMOs—use the same provider networks, and they pay providers through a mix of discounted FFS and partial forms of capitation. Moreover, as health plans have widened their networks and developed point-of-service plans and direct patient referrals to specialists, their HMO products are becoming increasingly similar to the products of PPOs.

ISSUES: NOW THAT WE ARE ALL IN MANAGED CARE, WHAT ARE WE GOING TO DO?

Most intermediaries offer a mix of insurance products that provide more or less the same physician networks and similar medical management techniques. They compete on the basis of price to employers, customer service, and benefits to individual enrollees, particularly in the Medicare market. Most of the savings they have gained were achieved by cutting payment rates to providers, and those cuts have gone about as far as they can for the short term. These plans are coming under three new types of pressure:

- Although intermediaries have been successful in cutting costs, the savings have been achieved by one-time reductions in payment rates. Meanwhile, utilization rates are rising across the board, particularly as these plans have added new providers to their rosters, included different types of populations in their membership such as Medicare recipients, and added new products such as POS. In the latter part of 1996 and through 1998, the "medical loss ratios"

(i.e., how much money was passed on to providers) of many publicly traded HMOs began to increase. Yet cutting back on product offerings is not an option, as their employer customers are demanding *more*, not less, variety and choice among provider networks.

- Employers, the government, and accreditation agencies such as the National Committee on Quality Assurance (NCQA) are demanding proof of quality performance. Given the lack of provider differentiation among different health plans, it is hard for them to demonstrate quality—particularly quality as compared to that provided by a competitor.

- It is also increasingly difficult for health plans to avoid a commitment to treat high-risk populations, both because of such legislation as the Kennedy–Kassebaum Act and because often they are getting a large enough share in any one market that they cannot avoid treating the sicker segments of the community. If insurers cannot avoid expensive cases, their only option is to manage the care of their numbers in a more cost-effective manner without cutting quality. How to do this is a new adventure for virtually every plan in America.

As patients from every venue enter managed care, the question becomes: Which intermediary model is best suited to resolve the issues of cost, quality, and care management? The attempt to find such models is a key driver for the future of health plans and for health care in general.

FORECAST: INTERMEDIARIES MULTIPLY IN TYPE

What types of intermediaries will patients use? For the insured segment of the population, the mix of indemnity to HMO plans will reverse over this next 10-year period. For enrollees in Medicaid, indemnity Medicaid will become managed care Medicaid, perhaps with slightly better access to providers. The uninsured will rely on the same network of safety-net providers, who will survive with a mixture of state and local funding.

The net result of this forecast is that enrollment in HMOs will increase from 27 percent to 47 percent of all Americans by 2007. Combined enrollment in HMOs and PPOs will cover just over two-thirds of the entire American population (see Figure 5-2). Only the uninsured, a little over half of Medicare recipients, and a few upper-echelon

employees—those in our "high-end FFS broker" category—will be outside of managed care.

Health plans will spend the next 5 to 8 years in a constant flurry of consolidation, experimentation, and restructuring. Several dominant strategies will emerge by 2005. Most intermediaries will adopt one or more of these strategies, depending on the geography, philosophy, and availability of organized providers:

- *The case manager intermediary.* The case manager intermediary divides a population into the well and the sick and permits the well to have free access to virtually all of its loosely organized provider network. Its primary focus is the aggressive medical management of the sick, often parsed out by disease state. It uses a mixture of provider organizations and relies on the development of information systems to track the activities of its loosely organized provider network. The intermediary spends much of its energy in directing the activities of providers and sick patients. Providers are paid in a multitude of ways, usually on a fee-per-episode basis, but must meet or exceed several stipulated specifications regarding costs, quality, and patients' satisfaction in order to keep their contracts.

- *The provider-partner intermediary.* The provider partner allows providers to be responsible for the medical management of the enrollees. The intermediary takes on responsibilities for customer service to members, for marketing its providers' services, and for redistributing risk among its providers.

*Figure 5-2. Managed Care Takes Over from "Unmanaged Care"
(Number of Americans, in millions, in HMOs and PPOs versus FFS and uninsured over time)*

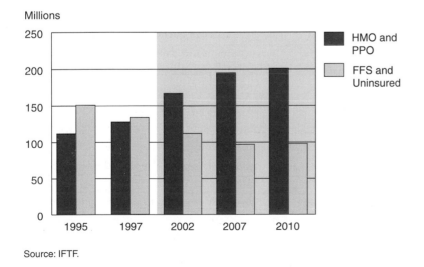

Source: IFTF.

The health plan relies on the use of various risk-sharing vehicles to pay providers, including full and partial capitation, satisfaction incentives, and rewards for customer retention. The intermediary rigorously audits providers to ensure that they manage patients to an agreed-upon standard but relies on the clinicians to develop protocols and demand-management techniques. This model operates successfully only with large provider organizations. Most intermediaries run this type of model in one region and the case-manager model in others.

- *The high-end FFS broker.* For upper-echelon Americans, the remnants of the old FFS system will offer indemnity insurance products or PPOs with very rich benefits and less rigorous utilization controls. Although these plans are unable to compete directly with the more aggressive "case managers" or "provider partners" on price, they are able to select better risks in their enrollee population and charge relatively high premiums for good customer service and access to high-tech and complementary care. Meanwhile, a slight majority of Medicare recipients remain in the FFS system, which provides access to a provider network that looks just like this one.

- *Direct to provider.* In a minority of cases, large employers in rural markets and a few big employer coalitions are able to bypass the major plans and set up their own administrative systems that allow them to contract directly with providers. The providers are asked to take most of the downside risk from these arrangements and to provide

medical management and population care to enrollees. Essentially, the intermediary functions here are shared by employer and provider alike. The financial solvency of this sector will not be strong for the first few years, but by 2005 a small but important portion of the market will be contracting directly with employers.

- *The low-tier safety-net funding recipients.* Most of the Medicaid population and some of the indigent will end up in a provider-partner or a case-management HMO, but some of them—and the majority of the uninsured—will end up in a "no intermediary, no luck" scenario with limited access to care despite the best efforts of safety-net providers. Figure 5-3 shows how much of the population was covered by each type of insurance intermediary arrangement in 1998 and forecasts what that will be in 2007.

REIMBURSEMENT MODELS: BETWEEN FINANCE AND DELIVERY

BACKGROUND

For patients with either Medicare or private insurance coverage, reimbursement for physicians and hospitals was on an FFS basis until the 1980s, when Medicare introduced a prospective payment system (PPS) for hospital inpatient services based on diagnosis-related groups (DRGs). The introduction of DRGs led to the early movement of Medicare patients from inpatient status to outpatient facilities where services could be charged on an FFS basis. Those outpatient facilities were usually owned by hospitals.

Figure 5-3. The "Fee-for-Service Brokers" Will Lose Their Dominance
(Percentage of population in each insurance model)

Where we were in 1998

Low tier (25%)
Case manager (14%)
Direct to provider (<1%)
Provider partner (6%)
FFS broker (55%)

Where we'll be in 2007

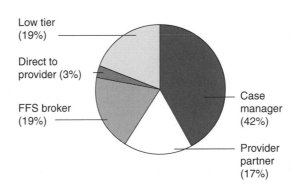

Low tier (19%)
Direct to provider (3%)
FFS broker (19%)
Case manager (42%)
Provider partner (17%)

Source: IFTF.

Meanwhile, in an effort to control the cost of health benefits for employees, many employers and employer coalitions moved to HMOs or other managed care insurance products. Insurers, except in staff- and group-model HMOs, slowly began to "push risk" to the providers, either capitating physicians only (partial capitation) while paying hospitals a discounted per diem, or capitating physicians or physician-hospital organizations for all required services (global capitation).

When we naively asked a Boston colleague why the HMO membership rate in Massachusetts was the same as in California, yet the utilization rates in California for all services were so much lower, he replied, "We have lots of managed care in Boston—it's just FFS managed care." The numbers in Figures 5-4 and 5-5 confirm that theory: the spread of managed care has not meant a significant spread of capitation.

In fact, only about one in ten dollars paid out by HMOs is in the form of global capitation—the classic Southern California model that was developed in the late 1980s. Although capitation is spreading outside of Southern California, it is generally used only for primary care services. Instead, aggressive HMOs have reduced FFS payments to specialists and hospitals and have placed money in risk pools that primary care doctors may share if their overall utilization and referral rates are below a specified level. The net result has been a transfer of resources from hospitals and specialists to primary care physicians and health plans without much global capitation occurring (see Figure 5-6). Many of the organizational models that hospitals and physicians have designed over the past few years have not been successful because they were designed to treat capitated lives. Even the Southern California providers found that some health plans

Chapter 5: Health Care Providers

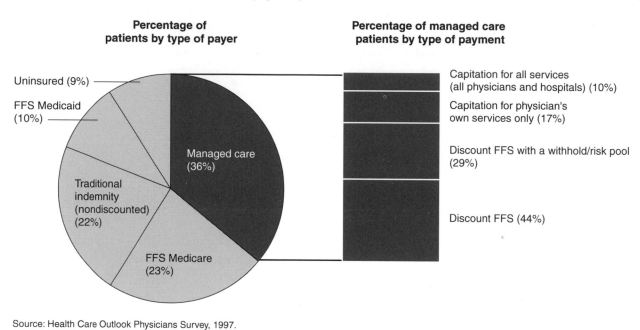

Figure 5-4. How Physicians Got Paid in 1997
(Percentage of patients with various forms of payment)

Percentage of patients by type of payer

Uninsured (9%)

FFS Medicaid (10%)

Traditional indemnity (nondiscounted) (22%)

FFS Medicare (23%)

Managed care (36%)

Percentage of managed care patients by type of payment

Capitation for all services (all physicians and hospitals) (10%)

Capitation for physician's own services only (17%)

Discount FFS with a withhold/risk pool (29%)

Discount FFS (44%)

Source: Health Care Outlook Physicians Survey, 1997.

did not want to pass the risk, and possibly the profits, on to the providers. Those providers who did accept global capitation found that the rates they were paid were restricted by the plans. When providers tried to resist those rate changes, they found that their market power was less than they had hoped.

ISSUES

While mixed payment methods for providers such as discounted FFS, withholds, and partial capitation on the physicians' side and DRGs and per diems on the hospital side remain the norm, they all provide incentives for more utilization. The health plans counteract this by attempting to control utilization externally. Although increases in utilization are still a significant problem

for intermediaries, they generally have not responded by passing that risk off to providers in the form of capitation.

There appear to be three reasons for this:

- Health plans that were successful in managing risk could be more profitable than those that pass it off in the form of capitation.

- Providers generally are not organized to take on the risk-bearing function of capitation and have little incentive to so organize in a world where FFS still predominates.

- Patients and consumer groups fear that capitated providers may withhold necessary care, although they fear that FFS encourages providers to overtreat in equal numbers. Several highly visible court cases have fueled this backlash.

Figure 5-5. How HMOs Pay Their Doctors and Hospitals (Percentage of HMOs using various methods for any portion of provider payments)

Primary Care Physicians

Specialty Care Physicians

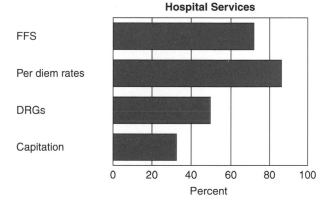

Hospital Services

Note: Percentages do not equal 100.

Source: Interstudy, using 1998 data.

The question for the future is whether incentives will continue for utilization and what the current flood of people into HMOs will mean for payment mechanisms for providers. The type of payment will have a great impact not only on providers' behavior but also on how providers organize themselves.

FORECAST

It is likely that neither global capitation nor discounted FFS is sustainable in the long run. FFS is inherently inflationary, and capitation raises fears of undertreatment among consumers. We believe that eventually a new way of paying providers will emerge. But for the next 10 years a version of the current system will develop that shifts toward more capitation because of the flood of people into HMOs. Global capitation will most likely double in prominence as the number of HMO recipients increases, but it will never cover much more than 10 percent of patients. Meanwhile, Medicare will start to introduce episodic prepayment for many of its components, including outpatient care, and increasingly will replace the current FFS system. Figure 5-7 presents a forecast of how dollars for care will flow to physicians.

Out of this mixture, a separate type of payment system will develop. Plans and intermediaries will devise reimbursement systems that give providers incentives to deliver care in a manner that improves quality, customer satisfaction, patients' tenure in the plan, and outcomes, as well as productivity and cost-effectiveness. We dub this system "performance-based" reimbursement, as payments will depend on the provider's performance on a string

Chapter 5: Health Care Providers

Figure 5-6. How Premium Payments Get Divided Up:
The PPO World Versus the HMO World

Note: These figures are hypothetical.

Source: IFTF.

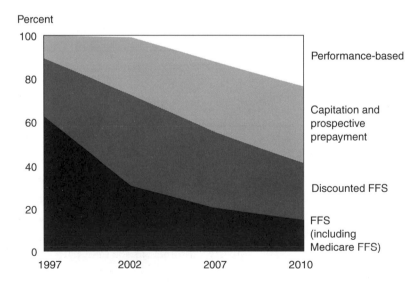

Figure 5-7. Fee-for-Service Will Fade, but Capitation Is Not Its Only Successor
(Share of physicians' revenue coming from different payment schemes)

Source: IFTF, based on data from IFTF, Louis Harris & Associates, Interstudy, and American
Medical Association.

of relevant algorithms. By the latter part
of the next decade, this system will be
the single most important way of paying
provider organizations, although the old
methods will still be a prominent part of
the system.

CARE DELIVERY ORGANIZATIONS FOR THE NEXT DECADE

BACKGROUND

The chaotic upheaval of the American
health care system that started in the
early 1990s is driven by several forces.
The most important of them is the
search for stability. Individual physicians
and smaller organizations have looked to
the large hospitals and health plans to
buffer them through tough times. Larger
groups and hospitals have allied and
merged with each other in an attempt to
develop bargaining power against the
health plans, which have also been merging to amass bargaining power over
providers. There have also been attempts
to change organizational structures and
processes in order to make patient-care
management more effective, but so far
that goal has been elusive.

Several types of provider groups have
looked to for-profit companies for capital, although the investor-owned sector
is a small, barely growing minority of
hospitals (about 14 percent) and an even
smaller minority of physicians. It does
not appear yet that there is anything
fundamentally different about the way
for-profit groups are behaving except
that the largest for-profit hospital chain,
Columbia/HCA, is backpedaling from

its national strategy. However, there is investment money available for people trying to create new types of provider organizations, many of them focused on disease management or specialty care.

ISSUES

Through all the activity of the past several years, most physicians who were independent have stayed independent and most hospitals have joined systems more in name than in terms of substantially changing their organization and governance. But the driving pressures of reimbursement reductions and the certainty that the challenges of tomorrow will be different from those of yesterday are driving continued reinvention in every provider organization. What changes this reinvention might produce are less certain than ever, and at present several models exist in different stages of evolution. They include:

- *Vertical integration.* A combination of providers and health plan, usually developing in an altered form of staff HMO (e.g., Lovelace Health System in New Mexico).

- *Horizontal integration.* A combination of several similar organizations, such as independent hospitals, in one system (e.g., Catholic Healthcare West, Promina in Atlanta).

- *Integrated delivery systems or networks.* A combination of physicians with hospital services and other types of delivery systems in one organization, typically by hospitals' purchasing physician practices but sometimes by physicians' acquiring hospitals (e.g., Advocate EHS in Chicago, Mullikin Medical Centers in Southern California).

- *Virtual integration.* A combination of various care-delivery services provided by separate organizations that offer services under contract to each other and are organized seamlessly (no good examples yet!).

- *Centers of excellence.* Single-specialty organizations that provide a defined service, either as a subcontractor to another provider or directly to a plan (e.g., MedCath in cardiology, M.D. Anderson Cancer Center).

The dominant issue for delivery organizations is which model will prove flexible, resilient, and profitable enough to survive the turbulent decade ahead. Intermediaries and end payers will demand not only cost-effective and efficient processes but also the ability to manage patients and coordinate care among a range of institutions.

FORECAST

We do not believe that any one organizational form will emerge by 2005 to replace the individual practitioner and large teaching/community hospital model that dominated medical care from the 1930s to the early 1990s. In order to satisfy the demands of intermediaries and patients, different types of organizations will use various models, each of which will provide a substantial percentage of care in at least some regions of the country. In the late 1990s, versions of each of these models are being built with more or less aggressive intentions by entrepreneurial physicians and businesspeople. They include:

- *The hospital-centered system.* The series of large hospital mergers in the mid-1990s were intended to create a model that provides all services in a metro-

Physicians in Group Practice

During the past 30 years, there has been an explosion in the total number of physicians in group practices, with an increase from 28,000 in 1965 to 207,000 in 1998—more than three times greater than growth in the overall physician population. What still surprises many people, however, is that more than 40 percent of all office-based physicians still deliver care in individual or two-physician practices. Furthermore, only 60 percent of office-based physicians are in group practices of three or more and, of those, about 70 percent are actually in small, three- to six-doctor practices. A practice of that size is probably too small to develop effective contracting and management skills during the next 12 years.

Despite all the press coverage and expectations, only 56,000 office-based physicians are in multispecialty groups of more than 100 members—the type of group best suited to accept global capitation. That is less than 13 percent of all office-based physicians and less than 10 percent of the market of physicians delivering patient care. Most physicians have not reorganized into large multispecialty group practices to counterbalance the forces of consolidating health plans.

Younger physicians, however, are more interested in group practices and other employment opportunities than they are in setting up their own individual practice. In a comparison of age-matched California physicians with less than 9 years in practice, the rate of practice ownership declined from 53.3 percent in 1991 to 42.4 percent in 1996.[1] Overall, between 1983 and 1995, employed physicians increased from 25 percent to 45.4 percent of all practicing physicians.[2]

Of this new influx of physicians into employee positions, most are joining existing group practices—they are not starting their own groups. These young physicians are looking for security. They will continue to swell the ranks of group physicians, but it will take time before they alter overall physician demographics.

The growth of group practice will not be driven purely by the influx of new physicians, but they will certainly be the greatest influential force. Our core forecast projects that the percentage of patient-care physicians in group practice after their residency training will increase from 46 percent in 1996 to between 57 percent and 62 percent in 2005 and will reach between 63 percent and 67 percent by 2010 (see Figure 5-8)[3] A historic shift will therefore occur in the next 3 to 8 years that will place the majority of patient-care physicians in groups. However, a substantial minority of physicians (150,000 to 200,000) will continue operating in solo and two-physician practices until 2005 and are likely to continue practicing that way, especially in more rural areas.

politan area across a range of facilities. The range includes inpatient, outpatient, diagnostic, and ancillary facilities, as well as physician multispecialty clinics, usually owned by or closely aligned with the system. These systems will employ many clinicians, either directly or under a contractual umbrella. Many of the systems will be based around AMCs, which will have problems making the transition to this more comprehensive approach, particularly in relation to their faculty and the physician practices with which they contract.

Fundamentally, the primary problem for AMCs is their organizational origin as inpatient care centers. The cultural inertia of the principle underlying the former system, which required them to "fill those beds," will cause many to falter. Nonetheless, in many areas of the country the large capital reserves of these systems and their significant presence in the market will ensure their survival. This is particularly true where their brand name (e.g., Johns Hopkins) is sufficient to ensure their presence in intermediaries' networks.

■ *The virtual physician-group cooperative.* This is an evolved form of the IPA—the most common current organizational form for physicians. Although IPAs originally were thought of as a transitional model on the path to "real" medical groups, they will continue to be an important factor to 2005 and beyond. Their ability to use information technology and their contractual flexibility to coordinate services will enable virtual groups to enter into contracts with several health plans. In many cases, the "real"

Figure 5-8. More Physicians and Many More Group Physicians (Number of physicians in group practice)

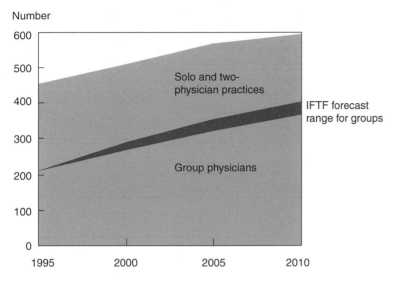

Source: IFTF, based on data from American Medical Association.

vehicle, the virtual group provides them with a substantial proportion of their patient revenue stream.

- *The corporate physician practice management (PPM) corporation.* The trail of for-profit PPM companies to Wall Street that started in the early 1990s will continue into the next decade. The main growth in this area has and will come from the PPMs that accumulate existing smaller practices, including purchasing physician groups abandoned by former staff- and group-model HMOs. While pressures from Wall Street will cause many of those corporations to fail, several will develop a common platform across their groups that is similar to the mix of corporate and franchise-owned operations seen in other industries. Considering the administrative inefficiency of most physicians' practices, there is no reason that these economies of scale should not show some savings. Achieving greater returns may prove difficult over the longer term.

- *The single-specialty carve-out.* In some specific disease areas, single specialty groups and networks of specialists will market their services either directly to payers or to other providers such as hospital-based systems or multispecialty groups that need particular expertise. A proliferation of networks will provide specialty disease management services for cancer, cardiovascular disease, nephrology, and AIDS (acquired immunodeficiency syndrome), among others. Some multispecialty groups that do not have sufficient volume will refer their patients in some disease categories because they cannot support nearly as

medical groups at the core of these networks will be neither large nor cohesive. The organization will be created from independent physicians with a natural set of referrals, on-call coverage, and clinical respect for each other. A management services organization (MSO) will help them make contracts with plans for business, with hospitals, and with other providers for services, and often will help them assume risk. The MSO will also help to identify and negotiate with providers whose utilization or quality is inadequate. IPAs will remain as an umbrella organization for these physicians, and within them there will be a range of activity, including attempts to build groups. Nonetheless, almost all small groups and individual physicians will find that, as a contracting

Chapter 5: Health Care Providers

large a specialty panel as can a single-specialty network. Patients needing specialty care will appreciate being able to go to these networks, which usually will allow them a wide choice of physicians. Some of these organizations will provide all comprehensive specialty services in a particular specialty area, such as cancer treatment, whereas others will provide niche support services, such as patient monitoring and education, that are used in combination with services provided by other organizations.

- *The remnants.* Changing an 80-year-old health care system that has been supported by government subsidies for the past 30 years is not going to be accomplished quickly. Some independent hospitals, such as profitable community hospitals in some suburbs and cash-strapped public hospitals in inner cities or rural areas, will not find partners or be incorporated into a bigger system. Many of the remaining individual and small-group practice doctors will still be doing what they have always done until their retirement. In that regard, much of the present system will remain in the health care system of the future.

MEDICAL MANAGEMENT: THE NEW ARENA OF ACTIVITY

BACKGROUND: FROM MANAGED CARE TO MANAGING CARE

While all of these arrangements on the intermediary side, the payment scene, and in provider realignment are continu-

ing, the number of people employed in the health care industry and the utilization of pharmaceuticals and technologies continue to increase. At the same time, consumers and physicians in tandem frustrate the attempts of case managers to significantly reduce utilization. Meanwhile, the health care industry has been rocked by the "realization" that it is the care of the sick that is expensive. Serious attempts are now being made to manage and establish routines for the care of the chronically ill in the expectation that this effort will save money overall, particularly in substituting preventative maintenance for adverse acute events. This is called *disease management.*

Because of the inability of health plans to control providers and the projected potential of disease management, control over the management of medical care will continue to develop as the key arena of activity—and conflict—in health care into the middle of the next decade,

ISSUES: A NEW IDEA MAKES SENSE AND TROUBLE

Medical management—active management over the full care of patients and populations—is currently applied sporadically if at all. The main issue is to what extent medical management will spread and be applied more comprehensively. In some respects this movement is taking the health care system from a state of managed care to one of "managing care." That active management component involves not only changing how physicians and clinicians manage patients, but also how health systems monitor and look after patients, including how much they encourage and support self-care.

The issue of medical management involves to some extent at least five parties: health plans, providers, employers, patients (and their representative associations), and the government. All of these groups are wrestling over decisions surrounding the creation of clinical pathways and protocols, specifically, what should be done and what should be measured. Intermediaries and providers are most concerned with control over adherence to those pathways and protocols. The main arena of conflict concerns who enforces the behavior of patients and clinicians: Will it be the intermediaries or provider organizations?

Still, the main question for the health care *system* is how much of the care delivered is actively managed. That question will be broken down in two steps that will categorize the population by their health status. How important will the management of disease states be for the acutely sick and chronically ill, and how much impact will demand management have on the generally well?

The most important question behind all the protocols, the process management changes, and the disease-specific approaches is whether they will make any difference to cost, care quality, and outcomes in the long term.

FORECAST: MEDICAL MANAGEMENT FOR THE CHRONICALLY SICK

Conflicts in deciding which treatment protocols will apply to whom will stay visible as a political issue during the next decade. Intermediaries, providers, and others, including specialty societies and quality organizations (like NCQA),

increasingly will issue multiple and conflicting guidelines. In addition, states and the federal government will continue to be involved in legislating lengths of stay for particular procedures and occasionally will demand minimum staffing levels and mixes in different types of medical facilities as well. However, during the next decade the focus of activity will shift from *designing* guidelines to *enforcing* their use.

Neither plans nor provider organizations will clearly dominate or appropriate the role of controlling utilization. For instance, the provider-partner strategy mentioned earlier essentially assumes that providers will take on that role, whereas in the centralized case-manager strategy the intermediary keeps that role. In either event, the prerogative of medical management will shift away from the independent physician. Both internal managers, working as part of a clinical team within provider organizations, and external managers, working for intermediaries, will assume increasing authority over physicians and patients in three areas:

- Managing physicians and physicians' organizations' adherence to protocols, guidelines, and pathways to ensure consistent application of best practices.

- Creating systems that extend care pathways across the continuum of care to all facilities where patients receive care—the descendant of current case management.

- Managing patients' compliance with their treatment regimens, particularly in the case of pharmaceutical use, and educating and motivating them to better self-care.

Whereas there remains great variation in medical practice patterns in the 1990s, the spread of guidelines will have a significant impact on medical practice and patient management for the chronically ill by 2005, and a sporadic but discernible effect on practice variation by 2010. Most chronically ill patients will be under some type of disease management program within the next 10 years, and there will be hints of measurable improvements in outcomes. The use of demand management by advice nurses in contact with patients via the telephone and the Internet will be commonplace by 2005. However, the struggle over who controls patients' and physicians' behavior between the intermediaries and providers, and among and within the different provider organizations, will not be resolved by 2010.

There will be ample evidence by 2005 that individual patient management programs for the more severely chronically ill will improve health outcomes in the short term, deliver more consistent and higher quality care, and save a small amount of money. However, there will be no clear evidence that overall cost savings are realized systemwide by the development of these programs, and their impact on the overall costs of American health care will be hard to ascertain.

WHAT HAPPENS TO HOSPITALS?

THE DEATH OF THE HOSPITAL?

To borrow from Mark Twain, reports of the demise of American hospitals have been much exaggerated. The growth in numbers of hospital beds stopped in the early 1980s, slightly before the move of Medicare Part A to the DRG-based PPS. Since then, reimbursement and medical technology have been pushing care out of inpatient settings. Beds have closed, from a high of slightly over 1 million in 1983 to approximately 850,000 in 1997 (see Figures 5-9 and 5-10).

The rate at which inpatient utilization of beds has declined has been much faster than the rate of closures, and hospitals *themselves* have closed at a very slow rate, somewhere between 30 and 80 a year, from a high of 5,800 in 1980. Despite all the rhetoric about the surplus of hospitals, not much has changed, and in 1997 there were still 5,000 of them.

So many hospitals have survived during what has been regarded as an unfriendly era partly because facilities and beds have been converted to day-surgery and 23-hour stay units, and staff time has been converted from inpatient to outpatient care. But it's also because closing beds and particularly hospitals themselves is very difficult for a variety of business, political, and social reasons. Nonetheless, hospital occupancy has fallen quite rapidly across the country since the early 1980s to an average of 62 percent in 1997 (see Figure 5-10). In the mid-1990s, even those areas that previously had been exceptions to the general trend started experiencing lower occupancy rates. For instance, occupancy rate percentages in New York City fell from the high 90s to the 80s by 1997. In contrast, some parts of California had already seen occupancy rates below 50 percent by the mid-1990s. Meanwhile,

Figure 5-9. Hospital Beds Are Slowly Disappearing
(Total beds in community hospitals*)

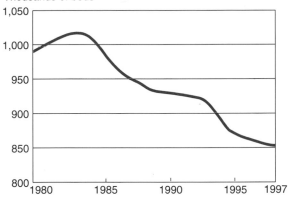

Thousands of beds

*AHA hospital definitions cite community hospitals as "all nonfederal short-term general and other special hospitals." This *includes* AMCs, for-profit hospitals, and state and local government hospitals that match the category. It excludes federal hospitals, long-term hospitals, hospital units of institutions, psychiatric hospitals, and several other specialized long-stay hospitals.

Source: American Hospital Association.

Figure 5-10. Occupancy Has Also Fallen
(Average hospital occupancy rates in community hospitals)

Percent

Source: American Hospital Association.

the increased needs of the comparatively sicker patients occupying inpatient beds have led to a significant increase in staff per bed over the past 15 years (see Figure 5-11). Rather than there being merely a *relative* increase in the ratio of employees to beds because beds were closing and those remaining in them needed more intensive treatment, there has been an *actual* increase in total hospital employees (see Figure 5-12).

Overall, the future of hospitals is murky. A combination of technological advances, managed care, and changes in Medicare reimbursement policy[4] means that the underlying demand for inpatient services will continue to fall. Community hospitals appear to be weathering the storms of the early 1990s by venturing into other services and reengineering their inpatient delivery services in a way that's allowed them to become more profitable in the mid-1990s. Average operating margins for community hospitals rose from 2.7 percent in 1990 to 4 percent in 1994, where they've hovered with little fluctuation since. Reported profit margins for hospitals increased from 4 percent in 1991 to 5.5 percent in 1996, only to fall off again in 1997. But these numbers are only estimates of true performance, because many hospitals use their strong investment portfolios to subsidize losses.[5]

Their larger siblings, the AMCs, are applying the same tactics. AMCs have been getting subsidies from the government, including DSH payments and GME subsidies, which have maintained their profitability over recent years. Furthermore, all hospitals are getting a greater share of their revenues from

Chapter 5: Health Care Providers   63

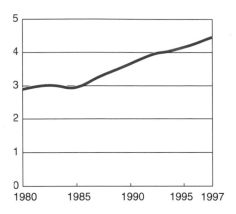

Figure 5-11. Sicker Patients and Fewer Beds Mean More Staff per Bed
(Full-time equivalents per hospital bed in community hospitals)

Source: American Hospital Association.

Figure 5-12. There Are Also More Staff in Total
(Full-time equivalents in community hospitals)

Millions

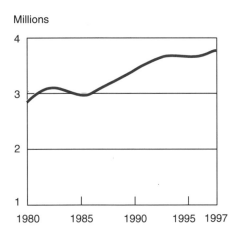

Source: American Hospital Association.

outpatient care and other services, and many plan to become more heavily involved in those services by making the leap from hospital to "health system."

The overall financial success of American hospitals is uneven—one-third of hospitals are failing, one-third are just getting by, and one-third are doing extremely well, particularly those that enjoy a geographic monopoly.

ISSUES

Despite the past 15 years of downsizing, pressures from Medicare, and the growth of HMOs and other aggressive health plans that have cut hospital days for their members, more than 35 percent of the health care dollar is spent on hospital services. That's a little more than the 34 percent they consumed in 1960, but down from the high of 41.5 percent in 1980. Moreover, hospitals remain a big chunk of the health care landscape: they are the biggest employers in health care and usually are major employers in their communities.

Among health care institutions, hospitals enjoy the greatest ease in raising and retaining capital. The increased number of for-profit hospitals, even though they still only account for 14 percent of all hospitals, has made for even greater access to capital. Hospitals and hospital-centered systems have been using this capital to buy physician practices, all types of ancillary providers, and each other over the past 5 years. But in the next 10 years some fundamental questions about hospitals will be answered. Most of them concern organization and ownership:

- *The for-profit, nonprofit divide.* Of all hospitals in the United States, 3,000 remain nonprofit and another 1,250 are publicly owned, usually by counties[6] (see Figure 5-13). But the rise of the big for-profit chains, notably Columbia/HCA, which consolidated

Figure 5-13. There Are More For-Profits, but Not That Many More
(Community hospitals by ownership)

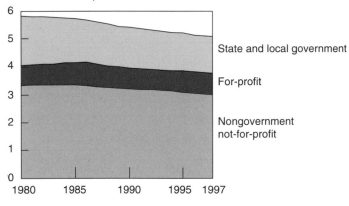

Thousands of hospitals

Source: American Hospital Association.

several smaller for-profit chains between 1993 and 1996, showed some market advantages for investor-owned hospitals. Consequently, several nonprofits began to convert to for-profit status—usually by selling out to Columbia. Only nine converted in the decade from 1983 to 1993, but 93 converted from 1994 to 1995. A combination of more aggressive regulatory scrutiny by attorneys general in several states and some bad publicity about Columbia slowed the trend in 1996. Currently, Columbia has reversed its aggressive strategy of acquiring and converting nonprofits, and the trend toward for-profit status appears to be slowing. But the valuation Wall Street has put on investor-owned hospitals is so much greater than the amount nonprofits can raise to buy them[7] that the incentives to become for-profit will remain strong. So this issue is not going away.

■ *The tax status of hospitals.* Though only a small minority of hospitals are for-profit, several studies have shown that most nonprofits act like for-profits in several ways with only marginal differences in their costs, the amount of charity care they deliver, and the way they deliver services. Furthermore, the fact that nonprofit hospitals—many of which own for-profit subsidiaries—advertise on TV, compete aggressively with each other, and otherwise look much like any other corporation is increasingly attracting politicians' attention. Given the tax advantages state governments bestow on nonprofits, might this status be withdrawn or amended in the future?

■ *The prevalence of hospital systems.* Many hospitals have announced or activated plans to become part of a larger system, even in the nonprofit sector. Usually this means a hospital enters some form of alliance with others; these arrangements vary from a nominal affiliation to full-blown mergers of assets—although most start with the former. Some 445 nonprofit hospitals were involved in some form of merger and acquisition in 1995 alone,[8] yet most hospitals still behave as if they were independent. Even in "merged" systems, there are often different boards and competing interests that don't look like a typical corporate organization. Some hospitals are taking an alternate track and staying independent. How prevalent will these systems be in the future, and what will they look like?

■ *Which services will be under the hospital umbrella?* The early 1990s saw hospi-

Chapter 5: Health Care Providers   65

tals trying to get into the business of offering physician services. But now most faculty practices have been "integrated"—with success akin to Stalinist collectivization—and many hospitals are suffering financial trouble with the private physicians' practices they've bought. Will we see a return to these health systems' offering only traditional hospital services—possibly employing hospitalists but not primary care physicians? Or will they be a base for creating truly integrated care delivery? And if they manage to create the latter, will they take the opportunity of Medicare PSN legislation to bypass health plans and sell insurance directly to individuals and employers?

- *The future of the AMC.* Over the course of the past 30 years, AMCs have increasingly delivered large amounts of routine care in addition to serving as centers of specialized tertiary care, teaching, and research. In fact, they have used their care services as revenue generators that subsidize their medical schools. They've also expanded their residency programs, both in their home-base hospitals and at other teaching hospitals in their regions. But this expansion is under attack on multiple fronts. Medicare, which subsidizes GME to the tune of about $80,000 per residency place per year, is planning to reduce those subsidies by 25 percent over the next 5 years. Moreover, while Medicare has been willing to pay the premium that AMCs charge to cover their generally sicker mix of patients, private health plans have become increasingly reti-

cent to do so—and have played AMCs against each other as suppliers of big-ticket procedures. As a result, AMCs are redesigning themselves. Many have merged with crosstown rivals to cut competition in specialty services. Others have developed regional health networks. Still others have struggled with a low-paying mix of patients and reduced state and local funding, and several are being spun off by their owners—usually universities—to other nonprofit or for-profit organizations. What will these battleships of the medical care system look like in the future? Will they be flexible enough to still play a role in health care service provision?

Besides the issues of ownership and organization, there are a couple of broader issues about the future of hospitals.

- *How many hospitals, how many beds?* We've seen a steady decline in the number of hospitals and beds. But declining faster is the number of occupied beds as more and more procedures move outside the inpatient ward. How many hospitals and beds will there be to serve the presumably sicker inpatient population?

- *How much money and will it matter?* Since 1985, a smaller share of overall health care spending has gone to pay for hospital services each year, apart from one blip upward in 1990. The money instead has flowed into home health care, SNFs, ambulatory surgery centers, and all the other facilities that have accepted the exodus of patients. Part of that flow is inevitable as tech-

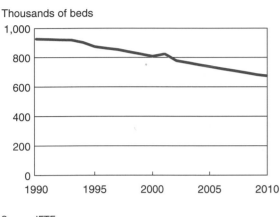

Figure 5-14. Hospital Beds Will Keep Slowly Disappearing (Total beds in community hospitals)

Source: IFTF

nology permits less invasive procedures. But part of it has to do with the intricacies of Medicare financing, which has rewarded early discharges from hospitals to SNFs and home health visits. Now that Medicare is getting serious about the cost explosion in these areas and private health insurers are increasingly putting providers at risk for a continuum of services, it may make sense for hospitals to keep patients in hospitals a little longer if it prevents other expenses later.[4] But the bigger question is: If we're moving to a system of more integrated patient care, does hospital spending *per se* matter as a separate category?[9]

FORECAST

Given the complexity of the issues regarding hospitals and their increasingly intertwined relationships with the rest of the health care delivery world, not all of the issues will resolve themselves

in the next 10 years. Generally, we do not expect radical change in terms of either mass hospital closures or significantly less money spent on inpatient services. This will be more a period of gradual attrition. But eventually the number and organization of hospitals will look quite different.

Hospitals and beds will continue to close, but not much faster than the slow pace we're currently seeing. Beds will close a little faster than hospitals, with occupancy rates falling faster still. For example, hospitals will close beds at a faster rate in the next 5 years than they will thereafter—our forecast is about 2 percent of all beds closing each year from a 1997 level of 850,000. By 2002 there will be roughly 777,000 beds and there will still be more than 670,000 in 2010 (see Figure 5-14). Hospitals themselves will close much more slowly. Even if they close at twice the rate at which they've been closing for the past 15 years, there will still be 4,300 hospitals in the year 2010; the actual number will probably be closer to 4,500. This rate in part reflects the difficulty of closing the big white building and in part reflects a transformation of many to smaller, more patient-centered facilities. Hospitals will still perform most of their activities without using their inpatient beds. However, in the very long run, many hospital systems will hang on to their bed licenses, waiting for the baby boomers to supply the demand for inpatient care after 2015.

In terms of ownership, about 1,000 hospitals will remain city-, county-, or state-owned facilities (down from 1,300 now), and about 2,400 will be traditional independent nonprofits (mostly community or religion based). The tax status of nonprofits will come into debate but is unlikely to change significantly. A minority—about 300 over 10 years—will convert to for-profit status in order to gain better access to capital, leaving about 25 percent as for-profit hospitals (1,100) by the year 2010. But most hospitals will stay nonprofit because of their religious mission, increased scrutiny from regulators about those conversions, and eventually waning interest from Wall Street in investing capital in an industry that cannot easily create fast growth in earnings.

Tracking hospitals' membership in systems is very complex, and several different definitions of "hospital system" will make the rounds over the next few years. But the AHA will likely count individual hospitals, and their owners will at least try to make them look independent and community based. So the official figures will look something like the Department of Labor's counting of "firms" and "establishments" where one firm can encompass many establishments. We estimate that around 35 percent of hospitals are currently in a multihospital system that shares a common overseeing board if not common ownership. This is likely to increase to 60 percent by 2002. As this happens, there will be continual increases in the sizes of various systems, particularly on a regional basis. However, by the time the merger and consolidation wave plays out it's likely that several will have fallen apart, and the number of hospitals in systems will be back down to 50 percent

or lower by 2007. The majority of the systems that exist after 2005 will be more "real" than virtual and more corporate: a single management structure will have final authority over the activities of all its hospital facilities—including the authority to close them down.

A similar pattern will play out as hospitals move into other services. Most will continue to be in the business of ancillary services such as providing home health care. Most hospitals will retain arm's length relationships with other services, especially those provided by physicians. A minority of the systems will become successful long-term employers of virtually all their doctors. Most will enter into looser relationships with virtual medical groups, single-specialty groups, and individual physicians. The pattern will vary greatly depending on the region, with more successful hospital-based integration with physicians in the Midwest and South than in the West or Northeast but with intense variation within each region. Successful integrated systems in regions outside of the large metropolitan areas in the West and Northeast will have the best chance of successfully starting PSNs and providing insurance coverage direct to employers—becoming the truly vertically integrated system. But the hospital-based system going direct to employers will remain a minority, even in regions where hospitals remain dominant as compared to medical groups and health plans.

AMCs will continue to face financial pressure from all angles. In response, they will continue to merge or at least will find ways to reduce local and regional competition in tertiary and quaternary care and extreme subspecialty procedures like transplants. They will face slow but steady reductions in their Medicare GME subsidies and increasingly will be forced to withdraw residents from other teaching hospitals. The problem of uncompensated care will increase, and the margins earned on Medicare will decrease, especially for outpatient services. But the political strength of the major AMCs means that they will continue to receive reimbursement from Medicare that reflects their mix of sicker patients. It's unlikely that many will take any option other than merging clinical services with their neighbors, but some may look to enter for-profit chains, and the possibility of severe downsizing or even bankruptcy will exist for a few. Those that are in the

public sector and have the worst payer mix—those with a high HMO penetration in their region and situated in a poor inner-city area—are the most likely not to survive.

In terms of overall spending—their share of the health economy—hospital services will stabilize at approximately 32 percent of health spending after 2002, falling from the current level of 34 percent. That will come as a combination of more aggressive health plans and the new lower Medicare reimbursements squeeze the rate of spending increases. Since the early 1980s, hospital costs have increased at just under 1 percent less than growth in total national health spending, and we expect that pattern to resume by the early part of the next decade. Total spending will increase from around $424 billion in 2000 to $560 billion in 2005 and $660 billion in 2008 (see Figure 5-15). By 2010, hospital spending will be about 30 percent of NHE, but the distinction between hospital services and other classifications will become increasingly irrelevant as some care is reintegrated into hospital facilities from nursing homes and other facilities.

The underlying change in technology—especially interventions and pharmaceuticals that reduce length of stay and admissions—means that inpatient days will drop continually. That's the main story for hospital services over the next 13 years, as it has been for the past 13.

Figure 5-15. Hospital Spending—Still a Big Deal, but Proportionately Falling Slowly (Spending on hospital services 1980 to 2010 as a percentage of all health spending and in nominal dollars)

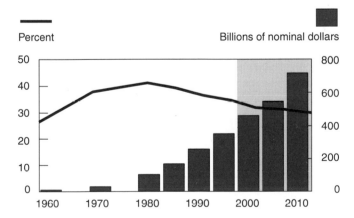

Source: IFTF; Health Care Financing Administration.

Wild Cards

- Physicians leave *en masse,* either retiring at an accelerated rate or finding opportunities outside of medical practice. The physician surplus disappears, and the clout that health plans have over suppliers evaporates.

- The consumer revolt against the HMOs and their descendants reaches fever pitch. Employers back down, leaving most Americans in a Cadillac-style top-tier plan, which doesn't enforce change on a recalcitrant delivery system.

- Medical management proves to be easier than we thought. After some research, clinicians identify what are the right courses of action for virtually all disease states and use information technology—enabled care processes to quickly ensure the best practice of care for most people. Practice variations decrease dramatically and outcomes improve considerably, resulting in measurable savings for the system by 2010.

- A new edition of the North American Free Trade Agreement (NAFTA), including the recognition of foreign medical degrees and residency training, allows the entry of some 100,000 Mexican, South American, and Canadian physicians. Supply is so great that patients, plans, and government take advantage of the newly available medical talent and seek care at lower prices with emphasis on better patient service. The privileged position of the physician in American culture fades.

- PSNs and direct-to-employer strategies work and take up a considerable market share.

- New epidemics and new diseases require more hospital beds.

- Hospitals become supplier parts of truly integrated systems. Their management closes facilities and beds quickly. The supply of inpatient beds reaches market equilibrium by 2005.

ENDNOTES

[1] Burdi, M., and Baker, L. Unpublished 1996 survey of California physicians compared with age-matched cohorts of physicians, extracted from the 1991 Robert Wood Johnson Survey of Young Physicians.

[2] *AMA News* (January 20) 1997; 40:3.

[3] This forecast assumes that there is no change in the current number of residents, and that all physicians retire at the same rate, regardless of whether they are in an individual, a two-doctor, or a group practice. The lower estimate assumes that all new patient-care physicians will enter group practice and that the number of hospital staff does not increase substantially but rather is consistently replaced. The upper estimate further assumes that 10 percent of the physicians in individual and two-doctor practices join group practices over the next 7 years.

[4] Reinhardt, U. Spending more through cost control: Our obsessive quest to gut the hospital. *Health Affairs* 1996; 15:2.

[5] Levitt, L., et al. *Trends and Indicators in the Changing Health Care Marketplace Chartbook.* Menlo Park, CA: The Henry J. Kaiser Family Foundation, August 1998.

[6] 1995 data from *AHA Hospital Statistics,* 1996.

[7] Johnson, R. Nonprofit hospitals: bargain prices? Letter to *Health Affairs* (July/August) 1997; 16:4. Describes why conversions make sense from Wall Street's perspective.

[8] Hollis, S. Strategic and economic factors in the hospital conversion process. *Health Affairs* (March/April) 1997; 16:2.

[9] The Congressional Budget Office clearly doesn't think so and declined to make projections on hospital spending in its 1997 forecast.

CHAPTER 6

Health Care Workforce
Future Supply and Demand

Despite unending speculation about the evolving structure of health care services, there has been little fundamental change in the way health professionals are organized and the way they interact with each other. For physicians, the number and variety of contractual arrangements has increased significantly, as has the oversight from intermediaries in terms of utilization review. But there has been little change in the way most physicians practice medicine. Furthermore, physicians remain the central figures in American health care with nonphysician providers poised to play a more critical part in the delivery of health care services but as yet unable to significantly penetrate the system. Although NPs, PAs, and other health care providers may possess skills that appear to be well suited to the demands of an environment with a greater focus on cost containment and managing health behaviors, their roles have been limited by their small numbers and the still significant clout of the medical profession. However, changes in the relative supply of new providers and their emerging roles may alter the landscape more drastically over the next 10 to 15 years than has occurred in the past 30 years. These changes in many ways will determine how quickly and in what way new service delivery forms develop in the future.

PHYSICIANS

Roughly 170,000 physicians are currently in medical training, with 16,000 new students graduating from medical school every year (see Figure 6-1). Adding international medical graduates (IMGs) to this equation, the physician pipeline is spewing out close to 23,000 physicians from residency and fellowship programs every year. Given that approximately 75 percent of IMGs remain to practice in the United States and that 7 percent of physicians choose administrative and research careers, an estimated 19,500 new physicians enter patient care each year. Over the next decade, the number of retirees is expected to increase from an estimated 8,000 to 13,000 annually, leaving a net annual increase of between 11,000 and 6,000 in the number of practicing physicians.

Assuming there is no change in the current production of physicians, and barring significant immigration or other policy changes, this influx will increase the supply of nonfederal patient-care physicians from 450,000 to 600,000 by 2010, or 219 physicians (excluding residents and interns) per 100,000 population (see Figure 6-2). Assuming historical patterns of specialty choice in which 70 percent of trainees enter specialties, the specialist-to-population ratio

Figure 6-1. Physicians in the Pipeline

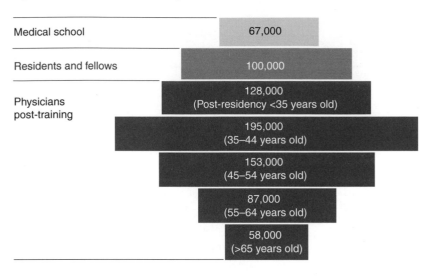

Medical school	67,000
Residents and fellows	100,000
Physicians post-training	128,000 (Post-residency <35 years old)
	195,000 (35–44 years old)
	153,000 (45–54 years old)
	87,000 (55–64 years old)
	58,000 (>65 years old)

Source: IFTF; Association of American Medical Colleges, 1997; American Medical Association, 1996.

Figure 6-2. In Excess: Physician Supply and Estimated Requirement (Including residents and interns)

Total supply of nonfederal patient-care physicians

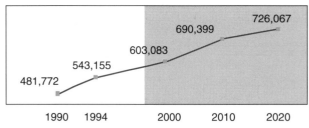

Nonfederal patient-care physicians per 100,000 civilian population

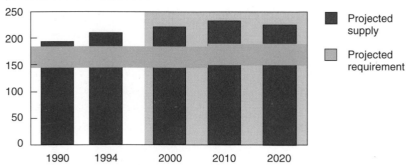

Source: IFTF; Bureau of Health Professionals, American Medical Association, Council on Graduate Medical Education.

is expected to reach 152 per 100,000 population in 2010, whereas the generalist physician-to-population ratio will remain stable at 67 per 100,000.

WHY SO MANY DOCTORS?

Over the past 25 years, the patient-care physician-to-population ratio has increased 65 percent from 115 to 190 physicians per 100,000 population, with specialists increasing from 56 to 123 per 100,000 population. Several factors have contributed to the growth in physician supply. In 1970, amid dire predictions of a physician shortage, the federal government provided financial incentives to medical schools to expand their capacity and foster the immigration of physicians trained in foreign medical schools. Between 1970 and 1994, the number of medical students educated in the United States grew by 65 percent and the number of residents increased by approximately 100 percent. However, when the shortage threat dissipated, not all policies were adjusted accordingly. From 1988 to 1994, although the annual number of medical school graduates in the United States remained flat, the number of residency positions increased by more than 80 percent. As a result, there are now 1.45 first-year residency positions for every medical graduate. The excess positions have been filled by IMGs.

DO WE NEED ALL THESE PHYSICIANS?

Even the American Medical Association (AMA), that stalwart defender of physicians' autonomy, has recognized that the United States faces an excessive supply of physicians—particularly of specialists, and especially in urban areas—and agrees that the unfettered production of more physicians is not the solution.

How does the supply of physicians compare to the projected needs of the population? Pooling results of four different requirement models, the Council on Graduate Medical Education (COGME) estimates that in the year 2000 the United States will need 145 to 185 physicians providing patient care per 100,000 population: 60 to 80 generalists and 85 to 105 specialists (see Table 6-1). Looking out further, a need for all types of physicians will increase moderately, reaching between 150 to 190 per 100,000 population in 2010. Each of these models assumes varying levels of managed care penetration (between 20 and 66 percent), various generalist-to-specialist staffing ratios (based on staff- and group-model HMOs, which vary from 88:50 to 56:81), and current patterns of utilization.

The main differences in the projected requirements are for specialists, as each model assumes a slightly different competitive environment in the future. However, even the highest estimates of specialist demand lie well below the projected supply of 152 per 100,000 population. The situation for primary care physicians is a little less clear. The number of generalist patient-care physicians is expected to remain stable at 67 per 100,000, a number sufficient in some scenarios but inadequate in others. With some specialists providing more primary care (see below) and the slowdown in primary care as a gatekeeper in managed care, we forecast an adequate supply of primary care providers through 2010.

The apparent oversupply of physicians prompts questions regarding the appropriateness of current medical education policy, particularly at the graduate level. Many advocate that the number of residents trained in the United States should be reduced to give preference to graduates of American medical schools. In 1999, the Pew Health Professions Commission went even further, recommending the closure of 20 to 25 percent of the nation's medical schools. But even if drastic changes are made today to reduce the number of new entrants, and new regulations make it more difficult for foreign medical graduates to practice in the United States, many of the physicians who will supply the future market in the United States are already in the pipeline. Medical training takes so long that any changes in either medical education or policy will not be felt in the market for at least another decade.

Table 6-1. Projected Physician Supply and Requirements for Specialists and Generalists, 2000–2010 (Physicians per 100,000 population)

Year 2000	Supply	Requirement
All physicians	203	145–185
Generalists	63	60–80
Specialists	140	85–105
Year 2010		
All physicians	219	150–190
Generalists	67	60–80
Specialists	152	90–110

Source: IFTF; Council on Graduate Medical Education.

Too Many Specialists?

In addition to being in excessive supply, there is an uneven distribution of physicians by specialty in the United States. Despite the shift to more outpatient care and the emphasis HMOs place on the role of the primary care physician as gatekeeper, primary care doctors still represent roughly the same percentage of all physicians as they did back in 1970 (44 percent). In fact, if we remove the primary care subspecialties and consider just general primary care, the percentage of primary care physicians has actually declined from 43.2 percent in 1970 to 38.2 percent in 1997. Why? Because, as Figure 6-3 shows, the money still goes to specialists.

But the excessive supply of specialists is now being felt by young physicians who are finding it more difficult to find full-time jobs in their chosen specialties. As news of these market pressures filters through to graduating students, there is some evidence of an emerging trend toward generalist training. For the first time since 1987, just over half of all senior medical students entered residencies in family practice, internal medicine, or pediatrics in 1995; this figure increased to 54 percent in 1999.[1] Even if this proves to be the beginning of a trend and not just a small blip, it will still take decades for this new ratio to be reflected in the population of actively practicing physicians. First, it will take 3 to 5 years for these physicians to complete their training and begin practicing. Second, they will be entering a relatively large workforce where only 38.2 percent of practicing physicians are currently in general primary care.

Although the number of physicians *trained* as general practitioners is unlikely to affect the proportion of primary care providers in the near future, more of the specialist physicians are likely to be providing primary care. In a 1997 survey of physicians conducted by Louis Harris & Associates, nearly half of specialists reported spending at least 25 percent of their time providing primary care, and 22 percent of specialists said they will be providing more primary care in the future. Even though specialists are not flocking to formal retraining programs, they are following the market's prompting. The share of all physicians *self-reporting* as primary care providers was a full 16 percent higher in the 1997 survey than in the 1994 survey

Figure 6-3. Median Net Income

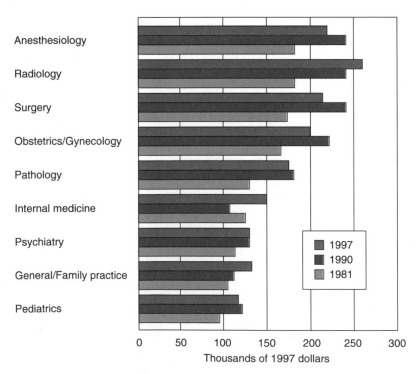

Thousands of 1997 dollars

Source: Association of Medical Colleges, 1997; American Medical Association; Center for Health Policy Research.

(46 percent versus 30 percent)—and we know this is not due to a large increase in the number of primary care physicians being trained.

The excess of physicians in 2010 will be primarily among specialists and predominantly in the medical and surgical specialties. The tragedy here will be twofold: not only will there nationally be an underuse of highly skilled specialty doctors, but also the money expended for a large portion of their training will have come out of the public purse. Basically, this is a waste of valuable resources whichever perspective one assumes.

There is the glimmer of a silver lining here. The excess of specialists may nudge some physicians to practice as clinical investigators, filling the ranks of a depleted cadre of physicians engaged in clinical research and the conduct of clinical trials. Others may assume new roles within chronic-disease management organizations. As the number of Americans suffering from chronic disease increases, these organizations will assume total care for defined populations of patients with diabetes, congestive heart failure, and cancer, and they will seek highly trained specialists to develop and manage their programs.

POOR GEOGRAPHIC DISTRIBUTION

Apart from the uneven distribution of physicians across specialties, there is also a geographic maldistribution of physicians across the country, with the greatest concentrations in large metropolitan areas. There are more physicians per capita in the more densely populated regions. As in any other profession, the cultural and social advantages of metropolitan areas make them highly desirable living locations for physicians. And areas with the best climates tend to have the highest physician densities. The more specialized the physician, the more pronounced is the maldistribution. For specialists, the opportunity to work in a large medical center and interact with colleagues is a critical advantage.

The issue for people living in areas with low physician-density is access to care. Not only may the closest physician be located several hours away, but the practice may be so busy that the doctor cannot take on additional patients. For many people, these are effective barriers to obtaining necessary medical care in a reasonable amount of time. In the absence of timely medical attention their health suffers accordingly.

Financial incentives have had a very limited effect in attracting physicians to rural areas where the professional isolation, long working hours (especially for on-call duties), and cultural isolation have acted as strong deterrents. In fact, the number of areas in the United States with physician shortages is greater now than it was 30 years ago. The most successful efforts to retain physicians have actually relocated GME training to these underserved communities. Once trained in these areas, physicians are more likely to stay and practice, regardless of where they went to medical school.

Medicare's decision to reimburse physicians for rural telemedicine consults will lead to greater use of this technology and will, to a certain extent, combat the professional isolation of a rural practice. However, the social and cultural isolation will continue to deter physicians from locating in rural areas, and the medical access problems faced by these communities will remain unresolved in 2010.

NOT A LOT OF DIVERSITY

In addition to the uneven distribution of physicians across specialties and geographic areas, ethnic minorities are poorly represented in the medical profession. Nationally, African Americans represent 12.6 percent of the general population but only 3 percent of physicians and Hispanics represent 10 percent of the general population and only 4.6 percent of physicians. The racial and ethnic maldistribution is even more stunning in regions with diverse populations. For example, in California, Hispanics constitute 31 percent of the general population but only 5 percent of practicing physicians.

Because of cultural and language differences, underrepresented minorities prefer to, and when possible do, obtain care from physicians with similar backgrounds. These physicians in turn play a major role in providing care to minorities, especially to those residing in underserved low-income communities. If the physician workforce does not mirror the ethnic and racial diversity of the population to be served, it is more likely that minority populations will not have access to essential health care services. In the absence of significant policy change directed at recruiting minority physicians, their underrepresentation in the medical profession will continue and will be further exacerbated in regions where

minorities are becoming a greater proportion of the general population.

NEW ROLE FOR DOCTORS

The New Inpatient Specialist

There are two new and emerging roles for physicians in the health care arena. The first is the "hospitalist" or "intensivist." These physicians work full time in the hospital, providing all of the care to the inpatients of office-based physicians. They are distinct from the radiologist, anesthesiologist, and pathologist who also work full time in the hospital. Most hospitalists are general internists, 10 to 15 percent are critical care doctors (hence the term "intensivists"), and 5 and 10 percent are family practitioners and emergency room physicians.

Hospitalists are perceived to be more efficient than office-based physicians, not only because of their greater familiarity with the inner workings of the institution but also because they are more capable of effectively managing inpatient care. Because they are constantly in the hospital, they are able to monitor patients more closely, which leads not only to the ordering of fewer tests but also to better patient outcomes. Furthermore, because hospitalists have the authority to discharge, patients do not have to wait for their physicians to conduct their morning or evening rounds—they can be discharged at any time, which leads to higher satisfaction and shorter lengths of stay for patients.

There is some question regarding the continuity of care that is provided when the oversight for patients' health is transferred among providers. In one sense, transferring the care of a patient to a hospitalist is akin to referring a patient to a specialist—and all of the questions regarding continuity of care that are raised with specialists also apply to the hospitalist. What is new, however, is the movement of this phenomenon into the arena of general hospital care and the transfer of authority for the patient from the primary physician to the hospitalist.

There are an estimated 3,000 hospitalists currently providing inpatient hospital care. Assuming that the average hospitalist can care for 15 to 20 patients at any one time and considering the need for on-call duties and time off, it is estimated that the smallest functioning unit will be four hospitalists caring for approximately 50 inpatients. Over the next 15 years, the greater efficiencies provided by the hospitalist will lead to increases in their employment in hospitals with at least 80 medical beds. They will also begin to work in SNFs. It is estimated that most nonsurgical inpatients will be cared for by hospitalists by 2005.

The Medical Manager
The second new training path for physicians leads to a business-savvy MD. Frustrated with their diminished autonomy in a managed care environment and intent on keeping an upper hand, many physicians are retraining, either in business schools or in health care administration, and are seeking employment managing other physicians. It is difficult to quantify the exact number of physicians seeking this form of retraining because many pursue this avenue through correspondence courses. However, as HMOs and pharmaceutical companies enter the medical management arena, they will be seeking physician

administrators who not only understand the health issues but also have the business acumen to manage their colleagues and their patients. The demand for these dually trained doctors will increase as forces trying to alter physician behavior realize that the best way to do that is to employ someone who is respected by physicians—and to that end, nothing beats a colleague.

NURSES

In many ways, the nursing profession is the most qualified to respond to current changes in the health system. Nurses' training focuses more on the behavioral and preventive aspects of health care than does that of physicians. Their skills are increasingly in demand in an environment that is moving more toward outpatient care and requires its health care providers to function as teams and assume managerial responsibilities.

REGISTERED NURSES

Registered nurses (RNs) are the largest single group of health care providers in the United States, numbering over 2.2 million. Hospitals are their primary place of employment. As the acute care hospital takes a back seat to other venues of care, one might predict that RNs' primary place of employment will disappear. However, despite the substantial rise in outpatient activity, two-thirds of RNs continue to work in the hospital setting. This ratio has remained steady over the past 15 years with only a slight decline since 1992. In fact, Linda Aiken at the University of Pennsylvania has shown that total hospital employment of all nursing personnel has declined, but the number of full-time equivalent (FTE) hospital RNs actually increased between 1984 and 1994 by 27.6 percent, increasing the RN-to-patient ratio by 29.4 percent. However, when adjusted for case-mix severity, the ratio increased by only 0.3 percent, indicating that the increases in RN hospital employment barely kept pace with the increased case-mix severity. Other hospital nursing staff such as licensed practical nurses (LPNs) and nursing aides have been reduced in absolute terms, suggesting that the staff-to-patient ratios for these nurses have not kept pace with the increased case-mix severity. RNs are providing more of the care for a sicker population of patients.

Although the average age of the nursing workforce is increasing, projecting greater numbers of retirees in the future, it is highly unlikely that over the next 15 years the current annual graduating cohorts of 95,000 RNs will continue to be absorbed into the hospital setting. The Bureau of Health Professions' division of nursing projects that the staffing requirements for FTE RNs will increase by 18 percent in both hospitals and ambulatory care settings by 2010 (see Table 6-2). But new employment opportunities increasingly will be found in nursing homes, clinics, and community health settings. Requirements for FTE RNs are projected to increase by 30 percent in nursing homes and 44 percent in community health settings between now and 2010.

The future supply of RNs is expected to be sufficient to respond to these increased demands although, as with the physician workforce, it will require a shift in training away from hospital skill sets toward more appropriate primary care settings, nursing homes, and SNFs (see Figure 6-4). There will be some downsizing in the hospital sector. We forecast a 17 percent drop in the number of hospital beds between now and 2010 and the closure of 13 percent of hospitals. This will certainly affect workforce employment to some extent, but we do not forecast wholesale closure of large numbers of hospitals, and an open hospital must be staffed whether only half of a wing or a whole wing is open.

NURSE PRACTITIONERS

The NP is a registered nurse who works as a primary health care provider, focusing on health promotion and disease pre-

Table 6-2. Projected RN Requirements by Employment Setting, 2000–2010

	Total	Hospitals	Nursing Homes	Ambulatory Care	Public/ Community Health	Nursing Education	Other
2000	1,969,000	1,231,800	128,200	134,200	364,300	37,800	72,500
2005	2,095,000	1,305,200	138,000	142,600	387,200	41,500	80,200
2010	2,232,000	1,386,100	152,600	150,700	411,000	45,500	87,400

Source: Projections by Division of Nursing, Bureau of Health Professionals; Health Resources and Services Administration; U.S. Department of Health and Human Services, March 1996.

vention as well as the diagnosis and management of acute and chronic diseases. Unlike RNs, 90 percent of NPs work in outpatient settings, one-third of which are private practices or HMOs. Although only nine states permit NPs to practice independently of physicians, over two-thirds of NPs have primary responsibility for a specific group of patients within either a team or a panel situation. More than 85 percent have the authority to prescribe pharmacologic agents. One in ten has hospital admitting privileges, and one in three has hospital discharge privileges. In some circumstances, NPs function as physician substitutes, and in others they serve as complements, providing health prevention, education, and counseling.

There were approximately 71,000 nurses with NP training in 1996, about half of whom are actually practicing as NPs. In the late 1980s and early 1990s, the expectation that there would be insufficient numbers of primary care providers fueled an increase in both the number and capacity of NP training programs. Approximately 40 percent of currently practicing NPs deliver primary care and 80 percent of graduates are specializing in this area.

The future supply of NPs will undoubtedly increase as the demand for their services grows and the number of training programs increases. Based on current training capacity, there will be at least 6,000 graduates every year. As demand rises, some of the nurses who are trained but not practicing as NPs may reenter the profession. Estimating conservatively, 125,000 NPs will be practicing by the year 2010.[2]

Figure 6-4. Projected Supply of RNs, 1995–2020

Millions of registered nurses

Source: Projections by Division of Nursing, Bureau of Health Professions, Health Resources and Services Administration, U.S. Department of Health and Human Services, March 1996.

PHYSICIANS' ASSISTANTS

PAs are health care professionals licensed to practice medicine under a physician's supervision. This new category of health care professional emerged in the 1960s, partly in response to the supply of experienced hospital corpsmen and combat medics returning from Vietnam and looking for work. In 1970, there were only 237 practicing PAs. Between 1990 and 1997, the number of new graduates increased 134 percent from 1,195 to 2,800 per year. In 1998, there were approximately 31,000 PAs in clinical practice. Approximately 7,400 students are enrolled in PA programs with 3,700 graduates annually, a class size that has more than tripled since 1990.

PAs' precise scope of practice varies across the country according to each state's medical practice act. They all require physician supervision, but in some states this supervision must be on-site and in others it can be provided from a distance. PAs provide basic health care services that 20 to 30 years ago were provided by the physicians themselves— and in many cases still are. These tasks may include taking medical histories and performing physical examinations, ordering and interpreting lab tests, diagnosing and treating illnesses, assisting in surgery, prescribing or dispensing medication, and counseling patients. PAs can legally prescribe drugs in 39 states.

Approximately 43 percent of PAs work in primary care settings, but there is a steady increase in surgical subspecialization, in which only 22 percent of all PAs currently work. Roughly one-third of PAs are employed in hospital settings, 40 percent in physicians' offices, 10 percent in clinics, 7 percent in HMOs, and the rest in nursing homes, correctional institutions, and federal agencies.

In 1998, just under nine out of every ten PA graduates were employed as PAs in less than a year. The growth in PA jobs is projected to increase by 22 percent annually between 1997 and 2005—9 percent faster than the overall job-growth rate in the United States. Based on current training capacity, it is projected that at least 68,000 PAs will be in practice by the year 2010.[2]

FUTURE EMPLOYMENT

In this cost-cutting era, health plans, hospital systems, and medical groups are looking at diverse combinations of providers as part of their cost-control strategies. The roles of many health professionals overlap to a certain extent but the scopes of practice for nurses and PAs most closely resemble that of physicians. To what extent will nonphysician personnel be employed in the future and in what capacity?

Staff- and group-model HMOs, which have the greatest incentive to employ the most efficient mix of personnel, exhibit great variation in their employment of nonphysicians, ranging from a low of zero to a high of 67 per 100,000 enrollees. It's therefore difficult to forecast future requirements with any certainty based on expected growth in managed care. There is evidence that some staff-model HMOs are using nonphysician providers as substitutes for primary care physicians, but this practice is not widespread.

Large multispecialty group practices and physician groups that are heavily capitated are another source of employment for NPs and PAs. The correlation with size suggests that smaller practices are unable to take advantage of the cost savings offered by nonphysician providers. Furthermore, even though studies indicate that nonphysician providers increase physician productivity and incomes, professional resistance certainly affects physicians' decisions. As an example, physicians are more likely to employ PAs, who cannot function independent of a physician's oversight, than NPs.

In the short term, the greatest impediment to wholesale use and integration of nonphysician personnel into provider networks is lack of supply. If all large multispecialty group practices restructured with a ratio of one NP or PA for every two physicians—which some capitated primary care groups aim to do—there would not be sufficient personnel to staff them. If training programs were expanded sufficiently now, it is possible that by 2010 the supply of nonphysician providers could increase to fulfill the demand.

However, beyond the supply issues there are several barriers to the widespread involvement of nonphysicians as direct-care providers.

- State laws somewhat arbitrarily limit the care that nonphysician providers may give by restricting pharmaceutical prescribing, requiring on-site supervision, and requiring case-by-case physician approval of services that are ordered. Organized medicine has a strong incentive to lobby and maintain such restrictions.

- The perception of lower-quality care, regardless of its merit, not only limits consumer demand for access to nonphysician providers but also may make health plans skittish about using them more aggressively in cost-cutting efforts.

- The salaries of nonphysician providers are approaching those of newly trained physicians. Although these income gains are the results of hard-won battles, in an era of a glut of physicians

and quality consciousness, medical groups and hospitals may prefer to hire a newly trained physician over an NP or PA.

Overall, we expect to see greater but sporadic use of nonphysician providers in the next 10 years. NPs with extensive primary care experience will compete with general practitioners in certain markets. Many physicians will still not be working with nonphysician providers in 2010.

WILD CARDS

- If only 75 percent of new doctors enter patient-care roles and 25 percent of practicing physicians leave patient care through early retirement, a move into medical administration, or a complete career shift, then the number of nonfederal physicians providing patient care drops to 432,000 (157 per 100,000 population) over 5 years.

- Americans opt out of managed care when policy changes in 2001 offer them MSAs at a considerable tax advantage. Freed from the hassles of managed care, physicians once again find solo and small-group practice affordable and rewarding.

- Although skeptical at first, patients find their experience with NPs and PAs exceptionally positive. Patients demand to see these health care providers on a regular basis; state laws are changed, allowing greater freedom from physician oversight; nurses assume key managerial roles in managing care.

Chapter 6: Health Care Workforce

- Frustrated by the power of large health plans and insurers, physicians embrace unionization. It becomes increasingly difficult for health plans and insurers to enforce compliance with cost-control efforts.

- NPs, supported by effective practice guidelines and computerized data on treatment protocols, replace physicians as the patient's first point of entry into the medical care system.

ENDNOTES

[1] Miller, R., et al. Graduate medical education, 1998–1999: A closer look. *Journal of the American Medical Association* (September 1) 1999; 282:9.

[2] Cooper, R., et al. Current and projected workforce of nonphysician clinicians. *Journal of the American Medical Association* (September 2) 1998; 280:9.

CHAPTER 7

Medical Technologies

Effects on Care

New medical technologies are one of the key driving forces in health care. From its unscientific roots, since the 19th century, medicine has made great strides in verifying the germ theory, creating aseptic surgical techniques, discovering antibiotics, developing anesthesia, and imaging the inside of the body. The impact has been huge: improving public health, extending our life span, saving lives, and heightening quality of life. The related cost impact has been equally large, especially in the United States, where new medical technologies are enthusiastically embraced as they become available.

Here we examine eight medical technologies that will affect patient care over the next decade. We describe the technology, then discuss the magnitude and areas of impact as well as the barriers to change where applicable. We've excluded some of the leading-edge developments that, because of the long lead time needed to bring them to market, will result in new technologies beyond our 10-year time frame. The technologies we focus on here are:

- rational drug design
- advances in imaging
- minimally invasive surgery

- genetic mapping and testing
- gene therapy
- vaccines
- artificial blood
- xenotransplantation

Even after a medical technology or technique has been discovered, developed, approved, and commercialized, it may take years for it to be disseminated widely. Similarly, in many clinical areas state-of-the-art knowledge is slowly adopted in community practice. We conclude with a discussion and forecast of the process of procedural technology transfer in health care.

We interviewed experts in many different disciplines and selected technologies that we think will be major advances evolving over the next decade. Although gene therapy is unlikely to have a role in the mainstream of medical management by 2010, by virtue of intense interest in its potential and a myriad of ongoing clinical trials, we determined that gene therapy will be a high-impact technology. In the eight descriptions that follow, we were selective in certain areas because a thorough review of the topic was beyond our intent of highlighting a particular technology for its future impact.

Additional Technologies

We conducted expert interviews to identify technologies that would have the largest impact over the next decade. The experts identified others in addition to the eight described in this report. We excluded these technologies from deeper consideration because, although they will have a significant impact on the health industry, their impact will be smaller or will emerge at a later time. These include:

- ablative techniques
- artificial livers
- cloning
- DNA sequencing/diagnostics
- functional neural stimulation
- joint replacement
- pain control
- regional perfusion
- tissue sealants
- treatments for drug-resistant disease strains
- virtual reality systems

RATIONAL DRUG DESIGN

Most drugs on the market today have been discovered in random screens of naturally occurring products or from analog development programs—once a time-consuming manual process. Today's robotic systems can screen millions of compounds in a year's time. This method of random trial and error is inefficient: of 10,000 agents tested, 1,000 typically show bioactivity, 100 are worth investigating, 10 go to clinical trials, and only one reaches patients on the market. Most current pharmaceuticals were chanced upon after years of this research by trial and error. Occasionally, researchers came across something that was not only safe for human use but also beneficial. The chemicals identified from these experiments were discovered as they existed in nature. Happily, we are no longer just searching randomly in nature to find therapeutic chemicals. Now scientists are *designing* thousands every day.

Rational drug design is the development of new chemical or molecular entities by looking at the physical structure and chemical composition of a target—a molecular receptor or enzyme—and designing drugs that bind to those molecules, turning them on or off. Drug designers use physical chemistry to identify qualities of the specific agent that initiates a pathology; once a known chain of events is identified, designers attempt to intervene at a particular point with a specific method. Designers use several strategies and methods:

- *Structure-based design.* The central assumption of structure-based design is that good inhibitors must be complementary to their target receptor. The two-step process begins by determining the structure of receptors and then solving the 3-D jigsaw puzzle of matching molecular structures by using specially developed computer programs.

- *Molecular modeling.* This technique looks at the physical structure of a receptor and creates the model of a compatible chemical entity by using computer imaging. This can be done with incredible precision down to the level of DNA coding. With the help of computed chemical algorithms, designers can build—first virtually on the computer, then "wet" in the lab—the molecule of perfect chemical fit.

- *Virtual reality modeling.* This is a form of computer-enhanced molecular modeling. It includes features such as a force feedback handle that permits tactile manipulation of a 3-D image of the candidate molecule model's orientation.

- *Combinatorial chemistry.* This technique allows drug researchers to produce quickly as many as several million structurally related compounds, which they then screen to find those that are bioactive and possibly have therapeutic value. The chemical attributes of those molecules are known, and the chemists working with them expect certain biological activity. With the development of more reliable and rapid screening tests, thousands of related chemicals can be tested in parallel processes for reactivity with a complement of human antibodies on a mass scale.

Rational drug design will shorten the drug discovery process. New chemical and molecular entities will get to clinical trials faster as the random and unpredictable time for discovering a compound by chance is replaced by these more predictable design processes based on the structure and complexity of the pathogen.

Because rational drug design may result in too many promising new chemical entities and not enough resources to test them all, prioritization and stratification of candidate products will be an important area of concern.

The Pace of Change in Drug Design

The pharmaceutical and biotechnology industries have enthusiastically adopted the techniques of rational drug design. Five years ago, few pharmaceutical companies were heavily invested in rational drug design. Today, entire biotechnology companies have been formed primarily to carry out structure-based design, and most major pharmaceutical companies have structure and computational groups as part of their drug discovery effort. In 5 years, rational drug design will yield a rich crop of new candidate molecules for clinical trials.

MAGNITUDE AND AREAS OF IMPACT

Rational drug design will have impact in a number of therapeutic areas. Chief candidates are:

- *Neurologic and mental disease.* Drugs are being created that fit the receptors for various neurotransmitters, potentially to modify nerve activity and influence the function of the nervous system in different areas where neurological and mental pathology are manifested.

- *Antiviral therapies.* Protease inhibitors designed to combat viral disease will be an important area of development. Every virus uses proteases to chop proteins into amino acids, which the virus then uses as building blocks. Targeting and inhibiting these enzymes could lead to the creation of the first truly effective antivirals. In the next 10 years, rational drug design will create antiviral therapies to combat diseases like human immunodeficiency virus (HIV), encephalitis, measles, and influenza.

KEY BARRIERS

One of the key driving forces behind rational drug design has been the increasing power of computers. The techniques and processes involved in rational drug design are highly information intensive and well suited to computer processing. The pace of drug design advances is regulated in part by the availability of research teams that combine knowledge of biochemistry with that of computer technology.

Unnatural Natural Products

Antibiotics that are in current clinical use are compounds made by antibiotic-producing bacteria and fungi—researchers have accepted the natural products that nature provided. Now, using recombinant DNA technology, "unnatural" natural products can be produced by combinatorial biosynthesis using genetically altered strains of a bacterium such as *Streptomyces*. Instead of isolating and testing a single natural product, thousands of novel biosynthetic molecules, a new class of antibiotics, can be obtained and screened. One such product may prove to be a powerful neuroregenerative agent that could be used in conditions such as Parkinson's disease, multiple sclerosis, Alzheimer's disease, and stroke.

Drug-Producing Animals

Transgenic animals can be engineered to produce proteins that act as drugs. These living drug factories can be grown from animal embryos injected with human DNA. Transgenic animals can be cloned, and an entire herd can be created in a single generation. A transgenic ewe can produce milk containing an antienzyme, and its use in treating asthmatics is now in clinical trials. A transgenic drug industry has been born as yet another product of biotechnology.

As researchers seek to combat more complex pathogens, they need to develop drugs that interact with their targets in more specific ways. With increased specificity and complexity will come increased costs in developing the proper new chemical entity.

As drug design can create an embarrassment of riches in terms of screened candidate compounds, much progress will need to be made in evaluating and prioritizing the candidates.

ADVANCES IN IMAGING

Imaging technologies present an enhanced visual display of tissues, organ systems, and their functions. They reveal the structural and functional aspects of organs, allowing clinicians to localize specific functions or conditions noninvasively.

Imaging has four elements: aiming energy at the area of interest; detecting or receiving that reflected or refracted energy; analyzing the data with computers; and displaying those data with technology that allows the clinician to view and interpret the information. Advances are taking place in each of these areas that will open up new functions for imaging technologies.

- *Energy sources* currently used for imaging include X rays, ultrasound, electron beams, positrons, magnets, and radio frequencies. There is a constant trade-off in the energy sources used: on one hand, the more powerful the energy source, the more deeply it can penetrate and the more detail it can reveal in the image; on the other hand, powerful beams can injure tissues and organ systems. The same ultrasound energy that reveals "baby's first picture" to expectant parents also can, at a higher energy level, smash kidney stones in an electrolithotropter. Energy source technology is advancing as scientists find ways to more narrowly focus an energy beam to avoid damage to adjacent tissue. Research also is being conducted on alternate energy sources such as thermal differences in order to minimize residual damage.

- *Detector technology* is advancing along two dimensions. First, digital detectors benefit from the trends in microelectronics toward smaller and smaller features on devices. The resolution of

Mini-MRIs and MRNs

An important trend in MRI technology is the design of increasingly smaller scanners with much lower capital and operating costs. The key: smaller and less costly magnets. Mini-MRI units will be available for dedicated uses in orthopedics, neurology, and mammography.

Magnetic resonance neurography (MRN) can identify the site of damage to a peripheral nerve by detecting increased signals at sites of nerve entrapment and trauma. It can also show the process of peripheral nerve degeneration and regeneration, the first imaging modality to do so.

those detectors is improving constantly. The first commercially available "megapixel" detector (able to detect an image that comprises a grid of 1,000 by 1,000 pixels, discrete elements of the image) became available more than a decade ago. By 2005, detectors that can resolve 6,000 by 6,000 pixels will become available. Second, there are advances in contrast media. These are chemicals that, when introduced into the body, enhance the contrast between light and dark regions of an image in specific ways; for example, by highlighting areas of malignant tissues or tissue abnormalities with more blood flow. Work is proceeding on contrast media that have organ, tissue, and cellular specificities.

- *Analysis of the images* is the next function in which there are rapid advances. Computer analysis of the masses of data from high-resolution detectors gets faster and better with increases in raw computing power. Breakthroughs in algorithms and techniques, such as neural networks, will speed the conversion from 2-D to 3-D images,

improve pattern recognition through better detection of edges and other features of images, and ease the manipulation and enhancement of digital images.

- *Display technologies* are getting bigger, faster, and cheaper. There is spillover to medical imaging from a range of applications that require high-quality images. Improvements include larger displays, higher resolution, richer and more meaningful contrasts, and deeper color.

MAGNITUDE AND AREAS OF IMPACT

Advances in imaging are combining in several areas. *Electron-beam CT* scanning—in contrast to conventional CT scanning that uses X-ray beams—offers substantial improvements over old technologies. It allows for rapid acquisition of an image, reducing the discomfort patients experience from remaining immobile for the duration of a conventional CT scan. While this technology can detect calcium in the wall of the coronary artery, showing atherosclerosis, it does not show whether there is narrowing of the blood vessel. With the development of new contrast agents, electron-beam CT will be able to show visuals of the arteries themselves, making this technology competitive with MRI, although MRI has the additional value of showing blood flow.

Harmonic imaging will overcome a number of barriers in ultrasonography. About one-third of all patients are "difficult to image," which means that a patient's body wall anatomy, for a variety of reasons, is difficult to "see" through. Specifically,

Positron Emission Tomography

PET was developed and applied clinically to the central nervous system for the diagnosis of epilepsy and brain tumors. It became the gold standard for determining myocardial viability and myocardial blood flow, but it found only limited application to other organ systems. Within the past 5 years the introduction of multislice imaging, 3-mm resolution, and 3-D resolution has revolutionized the field and made whole-body imaging one of the most exciting developments in imaging for the diagnosis of metastatic and recurrent cancer. For recurrent cancer of the head and neck, a notoriously difficult area to image using current technology, PET has shown an accuracy of greater than 95 percent in detecting recurrent disease. Although it is being used to stage many cancers, because the current technique uses glucose uptake as the marker, this highly sensitive detector lacks specificity. Within the next decade tumor-specific marker molecules will be labeled with positron emitters to provide more specificity, at which point whole-body PET scanning will be faster, less expensive, more widely available, and the most accurate and rapid means of detecting cancer that has spread beyond the primary site or has recurred.

someone who is obese or extremely muscular or someone with narrow rib spacing is often difficult to image. Smokers and people who have had radiation therapy can also fall into this category for cardiac imaging, and for OB/GYN a variety of impediments of the abdomen can cause difficulty.

Harmonic imaging improves the quality of images in these patients. Ultrasound generally works as follows: sound waves are transmitted into the body at a relatively low frequency and are detected by a receiver that is tuned to the same frequency. In harmonic imaging, the receiver is tuned to a higher frequency than the transmitter so that the clinician detects the harmonics, or the frequency-multiples of the echoes, that are produced inside the body itself. Higher frequency waves produce images with better resolution. Applications of har-

monic imaging include better prediction of heart attacks by allowing the clinician to visualize blood flow through the myocardium.

Functional imaging, which provides information about how a tissue or organ system is operating, will go far beyond the capabilities of conventional MRI, CT, and ultrasonography, which now provide only *structural* information about tissues and organ systems. PET has long been capable of metabolic imaging—detecting patterns of energy use in the body. High-resolution PET will offer pinpoint accuracy in these images, which will render many invasive diagnostic procedures such as surgical biopsy obsolete. Functional MRI is used to determine location of neurological functions such as memory and reasoning in the brain, giving us the first look at how the brain works. Future applications of functional MRI will be in the study of disease and the body's response to treatment—for example, changes in the pattern of neural activity in the brain of schizophrenic patients being treated with new drugs.

Because developments in computing power have increased image display speed and improved the quality and content of digital data, *image-guided surgery* is becoming a mainstream procedure. Image-guided surgery is a new kind of minimally invasive surgical intervention. It improves on endoscopic and endovascular surgical methods by allowing the clinician to see a computed functional image superimposed on the surgical instrument's location and other relevant information. The current combination of nearly real-time imaging and functional mapping will result in real-time, high-contrast, and high-spatial-resolution images.

Overall, imaging technologies will improve the diagnostic process immensely. Clinicians will use these technologies to look at the form and function of organs that were once examined only by surgery, reducing the need for invasive diagnostic procedures.

KEY BARRIERS

There are few barriers to the development of new imaging technologies, which benefit from the continual progress of computing power. Simple economics will limit the application of some technologies. Historically, imaging technologies have been additive—new technologies do not replace old ones but rather supplement their use. In a cost-constrained health system, more restraint will be exercised on the use of new imaging systems. Comprehensive analyses of cost-effectiveness, including the full life-cycle cost of the equipment, will become commonplace.

MINIMALLY INVASIVE SURGERY

Also called minimal or limited-access surgery, minimally invasive surgery was made possible by the introduction of fiber-optic technology, miniaturization of improved instruments and devices, image digitization, navigational systems for vascular catheters, and a sudden awareness that image-guided surgery was the wave of the future. Early examples of minimally invasive surgery were arthroscopic meniscectomy, endovascular obliteration of intracranial aneurysms, and

laparoscopic cholecystectomy. More recent innovations are image-guided brain surgery, minimal access major cardiac operations, and the endovascular placement of grafts for abdominal aneurysms. Over the same period of time, open surgery biopsy has been replaced by fine-needle aspiration of many tumors, which is gaining general acceptance for use on tumors of the breast and thyroid gland.

The movement toward minimally invasive surgery has promoted the proliferation of ambulatory surgicenters. The consequent major reduction in the volume of surgical procedures performed in hospital facilities has achieved a remarkable reduction in the length of stay, as patients having procedures previously requiring hospitalization enjoy more rapid recovery and return to full activity because of the lowered morbidity of the less invasive operations. In areas where minimally invasive procedures have replaced their more disruptive antecedents, short-term as well as long-term outcomes have been the same or, in most examples, better, with a high level of acceptance and satisfaction by patients. In the case of invasive procedures, less *is* better.

MAGNITUDE AND AREAS OF IMPACT

To begin at the top, brain surgery has been a major beneficiary of image-guided technology. Operations requiring access to nonsurface areas of the brain beneath the surface are conducted by using navigational systems and image guidance through small openings in the skull. Even more dramatic has been the impact of endovascular surgery, the creation of a group of innovative interventional radiologists. Using current technology—digitized image guidance, catheter navigational systems, and an array of implantable materials—endovascular surgeons can treat almost all intracranial aneurysms and many arteriovenous fistulas. Moreover, subsequent open surgical procedures can be facilitated by preoperative reduction of blood flow to the tumor or congenital arteriovenous malformation.

Endovascular surgery has advanced and matured rapidly in the past decade. The practitioners of the art fall into three broad categories with a slight degree of overlap. The first, interventional neuroradiologists, deal with vascular pathology of the brain and spinal cord. In addition to the procedures described earlier, these neurointerventionalists can lyse blood clots in cerebral arteries and veins, dilate intracranial arteries narrowed by pathologic vasospasm, and open partially or completely occluded arteriosclerotic arteries that restrict blood flow to the brain.

The second and largest group of endovascular interventionalists are cardiologists whose major procedure is coronary angioplasty. With advances in intravascular stent technology and the introduction of pharmaceuticals that inhibit the principal cause of restenosis—postangioplasty proliferation of subendothelial smooth muscle in the arterial wall—percutaneous angioplasty will further reduce the indications for open operations for coronary artery bypass grafting. Cardiac interventionalists can also correct cardiac arrhythmias, treat selected

cardiac valve disorders, and, by using improved technology, close congenital septal defects.

The third group of endovascular surgeons operate in sites other than the central nervous system and the heart; for example, they place endovascular prosthetic devices for the treatment of abdominal aortic aneurysms, create therapeutic vascular shunts, and perform angioplasty of narrowed arteries in the trunk and extremities.

Laparoscopy has truly revolutionized the practice of abdominal surgery for procedures on the gastrointestinal tract and female organs. The most recent addition to the laparoscopic surgeon's growing list of operations is bilateral adrenalectomy. Further advances will incorporate telepresence technology, which permits a surgeon to operate remotely, robotics, and 3-D imaging. Technological advances are proceeding with unprecedented speed, placing pressures on practicing general and gynecologic surgeons either to seek additional training or to drift into obsolescence with out-of-date skills.

Future refinements in minimally invasive surgery will expand the present scope and range of procedures. New arthroscopic procedures, wider use of image guidance in operations on the head and neck, and innovations in limited-access procedures for spinal and thoracic diseases are evolving; within the next 5 years they will be accepted practice. These advances will be aided by interventional MRI, currently used for liver and kidney biopsy, with its shorter acquisition time and 3-D capability.

For patients with acute stroke, interventional MRI will be a major addition to the surgical process. Pharmacologic brain protection will extend the viability of ischemic brain and prompt transfer to a dedicated MRI facility will permit immediate assessment of the brain's viability and blood flow. When appropriate, occluded vessels can be opened by endovascular intervention under the guidance of MRI. By the year 2010, large population centers will have "vascular institutes" that are serviced by emergency transportation networks. Vascular institutes will facilitate rapid movement of heart attack, stroke, and other acute vascular accident victims to an institute staffed around the clock by endovascular surgeons who can prevent the death and disability that current technologies cannot. Current gaps in ancillary pharmaceuticals will be closed by products emerging from the biotech industry. The development of stent grafts that can be used in cervical vessels and at branchings will extend their application at sites currently beyond the reach of endovascular technology.

Key Barriers

■ The American public wants big automobiles and RVs and minimally, or even better, noninvasive surgery. The appeal and marketability of minimally invasive operations have the effect of pulling these technologies into the health care system in advance of adequate technology assessment, including evaluation of cost-effectiveness. Adverse outcomes can and do result from prematurely applied minimally invasive procedures. The consequences could be restrictive legislation that would have the effect of creating major barriers to innovative clinical trials of this promising technology.

■ Insurers restrict or deny payment for new minimally invasive procedures by declaring them experimental and therefore not a covered benefit.

■ Currently, mechanisms for transfer of procedural technologies into the practicing medical community are barely adequate, bordering on inadequate. As computer-enabled procedural technologies evolve at an ever-increasing pace, their successful penetration into the delivery system will be restricted unless better models for teaching practicing physicians to use these technologies are designed and implemented.

GENETIC MAPPING AND TESTING

Until recently, most genetic tests have been used to detect rare and singular conditions. Many of these single-gene disorders become clinically apparent during infancy and childhood whereas others, such as Huntington's disease and polycystic kidney disease, are of adult onset. Genetic tests are used to detect carrier states and for prenatal counseling.

The special field of clinical genetics has evolved from observations of familial occurrences of inherited disorders to the use of the tools of human molecular genetics. Genetic tests have become available for more common and more complex diseases, many with onset in adult life. With the identification of cancer susceptibility genes and of genes

Chapter 7: Medical Technologies   95

The Ethics of Genetic Testing

When the importance and future ramifications of genetic testing became clear, a number of panels were convened to look at the technical, social, and ethical issues. The Task Force on Genetic Testing was created by the National Institutes of Health—Department of Energy Working Group on Ethical, Legal and Social Implications of Human Genome Research to make recommendations to "ensure the development of safe and effective genetic tests, their delivery in laboratories of assured quality, and their appropriate use by health care providers and consumers." The task force called on the Secretary of Health and Human Services to establish the Advisory Committee on Genetic Testing and to apply "stringent scrutiny" when a test can predict future inherited disease in healthy or apparently healthy people, is likely to be used for that purpose, and when no confirming test is available. The National Center for Human Genome Research has set aside funds for consideration of ethical, legal, and social implications of human genome research in which genetic testing has the central role.

leading to neurogenetic disorders including Alzheimer's disease, the Human Genome Project provided the engine that propelled the rapid identification of a wide range of genes that can cause complex diseases such as diabetes, cancer, and heart disease. These gene discoveries provided the basis for genetic susceptibility testing—recognition of a predisposition to disease—and with it unprecedented opportunities to intervene with strategies for prevention, avoidance, or modification of the predisposed condition. Abruptly, clinical genetics assumed a role whose importance was only imagined a decade ago.

No scientific discipline is as fast paced today as medical genetics. It seems that each week one or more disease-associated genes are identified and added to the genomic database to fuel a parallel growth of diagnostic and screening tests. To date, clinical tests have been devel-

oped for almost 500 human genetic disorders, a number that will continue to grow in the flurry of activity to complete mapping of the human genome

The National Cancer Institute has established three primary goals with regard to genetic testing: (1) identification of every major human gene that predisposes individuals to cancer; (2) clinical application of these discoveries to people at risk; and (3) identification and remedial attention to psychosocial, ethical, and legal issues associated with inherited susceptibility. A secondary goal is developing an informatics system to collect, store, analyze, and integrate cancer-related molecular data with epidemiologic and clinical data.

MAGNITUDE AND AREAS OF IMPACT

Genetic susceptibility testing for cancer of the breast, colon, and prostate is moving into clinical reality, and in each instance the hereditary pattern of disease provided the initial search for the identification of the critical gene or genes.

More complex genetic disorders, such as childhood asthma and late-onset Alzheimer's disease, suggest either a polygenic inheritance, in which more than one gene is responsible for the disease in a particular individual, or genetic heterogeneity, in which different combinations of genes produce the same condition in different individuals. Of even greater complexity are the conditions currently being studied in the emerging field of neurogenetics, where genes that increase susceptibility to schizophrenia, manic-depressive illness, and depression are studied to find out how they interact with nongenetic (e.g., environmental) factors to trigger the onset of the recognized disease state. In these psychiatric disorders, identification of the specific genes may give clues for designing pharmacologic interventions. The discovery of genetic susceptibility provides the basis for initiating preventive measures, whether through pharmacologic means or counseling. The new term "genometrics" has been applied to the discovery of a gene or genes responsible for a trait and to defining precisely the trait controlled by each gene involved in complex multifactorial illnesses.

Within a few years, our present methods of genetic analysis, sophisticated though they are, will be viewed as time consuming, labor intensive, expensive, and myopic in scope and application. New technology will use microchips designed to interrogate DNA or RNA samples for sequence or expression information. The chemicals for these microchips can be synthesized cheaply, rapidly, and efficiently by using the synthetic methods borrowed from the semiconductor industry. With fluorescent methods for the detection of DNA and RNA targets, hybridization will occur in a special chamber, and the resulting signals will be detected by scanning microscopy in a matter of minutes. Current applications of this microchip technology will revolutionize the fields of diagnostics and genomics. Within the next decade, cancer tissue will be analyzed for differences in gene expression, and in another 5 years specific therapies can be assigned to individuals with identified cancer genotypes. Tumors of a particular type will be classified by genotypic profile and, once

they are classified, even individualized treatment will be quite specifically administered. Applied to genetic testing, microchip technology will have predictive power for disease and disease predisposition that until now was almost unimaginable.

KEY BARRIERS

Practicing clinicians—generalists and specialists alike—lack the knowledge base to practice genomic medicine. Genetic testing, particularly the predisposition genetic testing for late-onset disorders in adults, requires a multidisciplinary approach. People seeking such testing need appropriate pretest education and genetic counseling and posttest follow-up care. Before testing is done, the person must be informed that other factors, genetic and nongenetic, may influence onset and severity of the condition, and that in many situations testing is probabilistic rather than deterministic. Potential consequences must be understood, as must the clinician's inability to guarantee confidentiality despite all safeguards and legislative protections.

Genetic testing has a predictable future based on technological potential. This potential could be constrained, delayed, or lost entirely through several possible developments: the desire in prenatal testing to enhance specific attributes of offspring; technology's advancing too rapidly for rational assimilation and application because of an understaffed clinical genetics workforce; premature availability of self-administered testing kits as a consequence of unregulated commercial interests; and ethical roadblocks imposed because of misuse of genetic information contrary to public policy (e.g., sterilization of people afflicted with a serious heritable disease to prevent genetic transmission to offspring).

With proper safeguards, genetic testing will revolutionize prevention and treatment of many conditions and diseases, but without these safeguards the possibilities for mass confusion, misapplication, discrimination, and lawful or unlawful commercial exploitation are sobering.

Gene Therapy

Two years ago, a blue-ribbon panel of experts sharply criticized the rush to initiate clinical trials of gene therapy before an adequate scientific base was established. The consequence was a slowdown in clinical applications and a return to basic research in several critical areas: better vectors or delivery vehicles to ferry corrective genes into target cells; more precise targeting of genes to specific sites and tissues; and enhancement of gene expression following entry into the target cell.

Nevertheless, revolutionary advances in gene therapy are preparing medicine for an epochal shift to an era in which genes will be delivered routinely to cure or alleviate an array of inherited and acquired diseases. Gene therapy can be defined as "a therapeutic technique in which a functioning gene is inserted into targeted cells of a patient to correct an inborn error or to provide the cell with a new function." The successful delivery and insertion of a functioning gene leads to the expression of a therapeutic protein of some kind that will supplement or replace a defective gene or treat the effects of acquired diseases like cancer. Somatic gene therapy, discussed here, only affects somatic cells—the kinds that are neither sperm nor egg.[1]

Current methods for gene therapy use directly harvested cells, cultured cell lines, genetically modified cell lines, and viral vectors, such as modified retroviruses or adenoviruses. In the *ex vivo* approach, cells from specific tissues are removed, cultured, and exposed to viral or nonviral vectors or DNA containing the gene of interest. After insertion of the genes into these cells, the cells are returned to the patient. In the *in vivo* approach, viral or nonviral vectors—or simply "naked DNA"—are directly administered to patients by various routes. A third approach involves the encapsulation of gene-modified cells and the reversible introduction of an encapsulated cell structure into the human body.[1]

A challenge for genetic researchers is to develop methods that discriminately deliver enough genetic material to the right cells. Most gene vectors in current use are disabled mouse retroviruses. Retroviral vectors offer the most promising prospect for the transfer of useful gene sequences into defective tumor cells because they target only dividing cells and have the potential of long-term expression. They are considered safe and effective gene delivery vehicles and are attractive because they are designed to specifically enter cells and express their genes there. Retroviruses splice copies of their genes into the chromosomes of the cells they invade, and the integrated gene is then passed on to future generations of cells. Since cell entry by a retrovirus occurs only when cells are actively dividing, this feature is exploited in rapidly dividing cells such as bone marrow but is not suitable for other tissues, such as muscle and lung. Unfortunately, retroviruses are somewhat indiscriminate and have been known to deposit their genes into the chromosomes of a variety of cell types, prompting research into viral envelope alteration in hope of increasing target specificity. The specificity of the envelope—how the vector is "packaged"—ensures the appropriate receptors are triggered.

Other viral vectors are also being explored. These include adenoviruses and adenoassociated viruses, herpes viruses, alpha viruses, vaccina virus, and poxviruses. Each virus has a potential therapeutic niche established by its attributes and behavior. The next most commonly used vector after retrovirus is the adenovirus, a DNA virus that, though capable of entering a dividing as well as a nondividing cell, has produced disappointing results. Adenoassociated viruses appeal because they cause no known diseases in humans and they integrate their genes into human chromosomes. But because they are small, they may not be able to accommodate large genes. Herpes viruses do not integrate their genes into the host's DNA, but they are attracted to neurons and may be useful in neurological therapies.

Liposomes are yet another potential vector under examination. These synthetic lipid bubbles can be designed to harbor plasmids—stable loops of DNA that multiply naturally within bacteria—in which original genes have been replaced by those intended to be therapeutic. A synthetic liposome-like vector, the lipoplex, can bind firmly to cell surfaces and insert its DNA package into cells at a significant rate. Mixing lipoplexes with DNA has become a standard technique for inserting genes into cultured cells.

Although currently undeveloped for clinical use, two new viral-based vector systems hold out the possibility of advancing toward the ideal delivery system for directly supplying cells with healthy copies of missing or defective genes. Both systems have the capacity to alter quiescent cells, such as the mature stem cells that generate the immune system. These viral vectors, HIV and simian virus 40 (SV40), share the preceding characteristics. Although HIV is a human pathogen whose use will be restricted at least initially to advanced cancers, origin from a human source may confer an advantage. SV40, an adenovirus, can be rendered harmless, is capable of infecting several resting and dividing cell types, is easy to manipulate, and is stable and nonimmunogenic; one wonders why SV40 has been ignored. Clearly this vector is not ready yet for clinical trials, and some safety concerns are unresolved. Still, SV40 appears to be as benign as any available viral vector and has the added attribute of being directly injectable into target tissues. Some investigators foresee the development of hybrid vectors that build on the best features of viral and nonviral vectors.

MAGNITUDE AND AREAS OF IMPACT

Scientists are currently debating whether gene therapy has definitively improved the health of the more than 2,000 patients in clinical trials worldwide. Current clinical trials are investigating the genetic treatment of several cancers and genetic diseases, such as cystic fibrosis. Gene therapy has succeeded in treating the symptoms of patients with hypercholesterolemia, and several children with severe combined immunodeficiency diseases are surviving as a direct result of treatment.

One of the most significant developments in this field is the application of this methodology to gene marking in the study of the biology of cancer. Close to 1.4 million Americans will be newly diagnosed with cancer this year alone, and the treatments currently available—surgery, radiation therapy, and chemotherapy—cannot cure 50 percent of those diagnosed. Although gene therapy was originally targeted toward single-gene deficiency diseases that are recessive and relatively rare, about 75 to 80 percent of the current clinical trials now focus on cancer.

For treating cancer, a variety of approaches are being attempted. Some involve imparting cancer cells with genes that give rise to toxic molecules. When these genes are expressed, the resulting product then kills the cancer cells. Genetic marking of marrow cells used in similar *ex vivo* therapies permits physicians to monitor the effects of different cancer-purging methods. Another research focus is on the correction or compensation for acquired genetic mutations, particularly of the oft-mutated tumor suppressor gene p53.

Yet another field of cancer research is immunotherapy. Immunotherapeutic research concentrates on how tumors evade detection and attack via the immune system, how they spread away from their sites of origin, how they gain a new blood supply, and how they evolve and spread.

A different form of genetic marking is used in immunotherapy, also called vaccine therapy. Immunotherapeutic vaccinations tag cancer cells with certain genes that make them more visible to the immune system. One method being widely tested involves modifying a patient's cancer cells with genes encoding cytokines—the communication proteins of the immune system's *B* and *T* cells—to draw an attack from the immune system. Unfortunately, this method will benefit only patients with robust immune systems and not those with advanced cancer.

KEY BARRIERS

Despite encouraging results, the field awaits answers to many unresolved questions. An area where enormous progress has been made, but where much more is needed, is developing gene-delivery vectors. Virus-based vectors have been the most efficient for inserting genes into cells in the laboratory, but in clinical applications the results have in some cases been short lived, and there have been unwanted side effects.

In addition, the field needs to develop animal models to test the biological and clinical efficacy of the new vectors and procedures. As a result, gene therapy may take longer to reach patients than originally predicted. The progress of gene therapy also depends on adequate technical, financial, and training resources, and demands close interaction between academics, clinicians, and private-sector companies.

Private companies are playing a critical role in promoting the development of innovative medical technology. They have millions of dollars at risk: they have to choose technologies, knowing that the ultimately successful approaches are likely to require complex assemblies of new chemical tools and procedures. For industry, a necessary incentive is the award of exclusive protection of innovative breakthroughs. Limited access to enabling technologies for gene therapy—such as vectors—because of time-consuming and expensive licensing processes, could lead to prohibitive commercial burdens that would delay progress in the field.

In June 1999, there were 313 clinical studies involving gene transfer, of which 277 protocols involved new therapeutic applications with most (193) intended for patients with cancer. The same advisory group that in 1995 accused the scientific community of overselling the present benefits of gene therapy stressed the extraordinary potential of gene therapy for the long-term treatment of human disease. The lack of more efficient gene vectors was singled out as the major barrier to attaining better clinical results.[2]

With the intense ongoing activity in vector development, we project that

within 10 years a number of efficient gene delivery systems will be in clinical use. Vectors that have both site- and cell-type specificities will deliver genes to treat a wide range of conditions in most, if not all, organs. The potential of using genes and gene products in novel strategies is an incredibly powerful incentive to pursue gene therapy as the equal of the future's most effective therapeutic modalities.

VACCINES

Since Jenner conferred smallpox immunity with inoculations of cowpox in the early 19th century, vaccines have been administered globally as preventive measures for acute diseases, such as diphtheria, smallpox, and whooping cough, and have been used to avoid acute infection by creating a low-level immune response that remains as an acquired immunity. In the history of public health, vaccines have proved to be among the most effective disease prevention tools. Some diseases, such as smallpox, polio, and measles have been eradicated or brought under control through mass vaccination programs.

The current use of vaccines includes any preparation intended for active immunization of the recipient. Until recently, vaccines were prophylactic—their sole objective was preventing a specific infectious disease. They were therefore directed against the causative infectious agent. Lately, vaccines have been used against noninfectious diseases. Patients with certain cancers have been vaccinated—either prophylactically, to prevent the emergence of micrometastatic tumors, or therapeutically, to boost the immunologic cytotoxic response to the tumor.

Vaccines can have preventive and therapeutic uses. Preventive vaccines permit the vaccinated individual to develop immunologic responses that prevent or modulate subsequent infection or disease. Recently developed therapeutic vaccines use new recombinant DNA technology to provide genetic therapy to patients who already have a disease. The key to using this technology is specificity for tumor cells.

The application of molecular biology to the identification of virulent genes has led to a fundamental understanding of the pathogenesis of virulent microbes. With the molecular tools of the new genetics, the genes responsible for the organism's virulence can be identified and isolated. The molecular genetic definition of virulence has exciting and highly promising implications for vaccines. Given the side effects of antibiotics, including the emergence of resistant bacteria, novel strategies for controlling infectious diseases are evolving. One of the most promising strategies, that of using molecular microbiology and whole-gene sequencing to develop candidate vaccines, will be the wider use of gene-specific vaccines.[3]

Recent therapeutic vaccines are designed to attack certain chronic infections. Early cancer vaccines had few successes but with the new knowledge and technology ushered in by molecular biology, medical, and recombinant DNA technology, anticancer vaccines are gaining increasing attention. This resurgence of interest in therapeutic vaccines reflects a new and broadened understanding of the immune system and its elements.

Vaccines have been effective in treating melanomas and renal cell carcinomas, two cancers that are unique in their responsiveness to the immune system. Vaccine therapies for cancer that stimulate the immune system and don't involve surgery, radiation, or cytotoxicity could become the least traumatic mode of treatment for particular cancer patients. A vaccine can activate the immune system by delivering a tumor antigen or by eliciting a nonspecific immune system response. A nonspecific response would simply boost the activity of the immune system, resulting in greater overall immune activity.

MAGNITUDE AND AREAS OF IMPACT

Prophylactic vaccination to prevent cancers caused by viruses would prevent an estimated 850,000 cases of cancer each year, roughly 11 percent of the global cancer burden. Examples of such viruses and their secondary cancers are Epstein-Barr virus and nasopharyngeal cancer, human papilloma virus (HPV) and cancer of the cervix, and hepatitis B virus and primary liver cancer. Because cervical cancer is diagnosed in 16,000 women in the United States each year, the impact of a vaccine for HPV will be substantial. In addition, a live attenuated HIV vaccine may be a realistic projection by 2005, or even sooner.

A novel new vaccine against rotavirus, a major cause of childhood diarrheal disease mortality in developing countries, that causes an estimated 600,000 deaths worldwide each year, is a live oral rotavirus vaccine. Incorporation of this vaccine into routine immunization could reduce severe rotavirus gastroenteritis by 90 percent.

Could some diseases currently believed to have a noninfectious cause be the direct consequence of an infection by an unidentified or unrecognized agent? If the recent connection of *H. pylori* infection to gastric carcinoma and lymphoma and the putative role of infectious prions with Alzheimer's disease are a prelude to the future, the answer is a resounding "yes." Among immediate candidates for such an etiologic connection are other cancers and rheumatoid arthritis. By the year 2010, prophylactic and therapeutic vaccines will compete with rational drug design for airtime.

KEY BARRIERS

Advances in vaccine development are contingent on the same obstacles that must be overcome in gene therapy— delivering enough of the immune system trigger and to the right cells. Vector development to increase the efficacy of delivery is what vaccine departments at most major pharmaceutical companies are working on now.

Clinical trials of HIV vaccines will undoubtedly be controversial and politically charged. Traditional approaches to vaccine development, such as "whole killed" or attenuated virus methods, raise special safety concerns with HIV because a faulty vaccine that actually

infects a recipient would have lethal consequences. HIV vaccine research goals may focus on a product that can inhibit progression to disease or lower viral load in infected persons instead of preventing actual infection.

ARTIFICIAL BLOOD

Blood transfusions are given for two reasons: (1) to increase oxygen-carrying capacity, and (2) to restore intravascular volume. Intravascular volume can be restored by other fluids, such as crystalloids and colloids, which are free from the risks of transmitting an infectious agent. Thus, increasing oxygen-carrying capacity is rapidly becoming the *sole* indication for blood transfusions, which in most cases is done by administering packed red blood cells. The only major risk of blood transfusion, assuming the absence of human error in the pretransfusion process, is transmission of an infectious agent that has eluded detection by the battery of screening tests currently performed before a unit of blood is cleared for use. The principal concerns are the HIV and hepatitis viruses, capable of producing fatal or crippling diseases for which no effective treatment currently exists. Availability of donated blood in the United States does not pose a problem, infrequent temporary shortages being geographically restricted and short lived.

Historically, the armed services have tried to develop artificial blood for military use under wartime conditions and in natural disasters. The features of an ideal blood substitute would be ready availability, safety, long shelf life, efficacy, and compatibility across all blood types. Interest in artificial blood peaked in the 1980s because of the seriousness of transfusion transmission of HIV and hepatitis infections.

MAGNITUDE AND AREAS OF IMPACT

Hemoglobin-free fluids carrying dissolved oxygen have been approved for clinical use but because of their inability to achieve desired oxygenation of tissues these products have not been used much in practice.

Hemoglobin-containing products have been produced by using outdated human blood or bovine blood. A serious drawback of these hemoglobin products has been kidney damage caused by the splitting of hemoglobin into agents that were shown to damage the kidneys. Human hemoglobin can be chemically stabilized to avoid this splitting, and refined blood substitutes based on human hemoglobin are now in advanced clinical trials. The obvious problems are the supply of outdated blood and the risk, although reduced, of disease transmission.

A new company, Somatogen, has produced a recombinant hemoglobin using *E. coli.* The recombinant hemoglobin acts like human hemoglobin, and the synthetic process can be programmed to produce a product with an ideal oxygen-release curve. The recombinant hemoglobin, like stabilized human hemoglobin, has a half-life of 24 hours. Food and Drug Administration (FDA) approval of stabilized human and synthetic hemoglobin products should have a satisfactory blood substitute widely available by

the year 2000. Further refinements of synthetic hemoglobin molecules will lead to a near-ideal substitute for blood by 2010. This fluid will have a shelf life of 1 year or longer; obviate the need for cross-match (i.e., be a universal source of blood); and carry no risk of infection. Such a product will be used routinely for cardiac bypass procedures and renal dialysis as well as for transfusion.

KEY BARRIERS

- Public's reluctance to accept an artificial product that is perceived to be less valuable.

- Resistance from an entrenched blood-bank industry.

- High cost of artificial blood due to manufacturers' need to have an early return on investment in product development.

XENOTRANSPLANTATION

Xenotransplantation—the transplantation of cells, tissues, and whole organs from one species to another—had its modern beginning in the early 1960s with the transplantation of kidneys from chimpanzees to six human patients. But these xenotransplants, and later other grafts of solid organs across species, resulted in immune rejection after brief periods of normal function in the new host. In contrast, allotransplantation—transplantation within species—of bone marrow and solid organs from related and unrelated human donors has become highly successful because of satisfactory, although less-than-ideal, means of avoiding immune rejection, principally by using immunosuppressive drugs and avoiding major histoincompatibilities to the extent possible.

MAGNITUDE AND AREAS OF IMPACT

The number of patients meeting strict criteria for receiving transplants of kidneys, lungs, livers, and hearts currently exceeds the supply of suitable donor organs. In the past 10 years, the number of solid-organ allotransplants has increased slightly more than 50 percent, with the greatest increase being in lung transplants. Over the same span of time, the number of names on the waiting list for all organs reached 66,000, in September 1999, and 4,900 potential recipients died in 1998 while awaiting a suitable donor organ. Median waiting times in 1998 were 1.3 years for livers, more than 1.5 years for lungs, and more than 2.5 years for kidneys. In 1998 nearly 21,000 organ transplants were projected: 13,000 kidneys, 4,500 livers, 1,200 pancreases, 2,400 hearts, and 900 lungs. Availability of a suitable donor organ poses a particular problem for infants and children because of organ size, and for ethnic minorities because of a lack of suitably matched donors.

As indications for organ transplantation have broadened, waiting lists grown, and waiting times for suitable human organs lengthened, research on xenotransplantation has accelerated by using new knowledge and methods of molecular genetics, transplantation biology, genetic engineering, and transgenic technology. Current xenotransplantation research focuses on the pig because of its size and favorable biologic factors.

The basic strategies fall in two areas: combined transplantation of bone marrow and the solid organ; and modification of the animal serving as the source of the organ. Both strategies are designed to avoid acute rejection. Combined transplantation, considered a high risk but an equally high-reward strategy, depends on first successfully grafting the foreign bone marrow into the patient, thus permitting later successful transplantation of the solid organ. The strategy more likely to be successful is genetic modification of the pig using transgenic technology. Introduction of a new gene requires 14 months, but this time will be shortened in the future. The short-term goal will be to use organs from modified pig donors to bridge a human recipient for a matter of months while awaiting a suitable human organ, and this may be possible within the next 2 years. The use of pig organs as bridges will teach critical lessons essential to the creation of transgenic pigs whose organs can be transplanted for permanent replacement, an ideal that should be attained within 10 years. Humans are presently living with xenotransplants of nervous tissue mechanically transplanted to the brain for the treatment of Parkinson's disease, so the feasibility of organ xenotransplantation is not far-fetched.

Transplantation of organs has been one of the great medical advances of the century and the one modality that treats a chronic disease successfully by replacing the diseased organ. The present limitation of solid-organ transplantation is the availability of donor organs, and for both social and economic reasons, current wait lists do not reflect the true need for

Chapter 7: Medical Technologies

organ transplants in our population. The applications of xenotransplantation go beyond eliminating the waiting lists for solid organs as they are now used. Chronic conditions, such as diabetes and Parkinson's disease, can be successfully treated with xenotransplants, and xeno-transplants of cells and tissues can be used to transfer genes and their gene products for the treatment of genetic diseases, such as hemophilia, and acquired conditions, such as cancer. Pediatric organ transplants could be used in the treatment of congenital heart disease and as a prophylactic measure in the patient with Wilm's disease. The potential is incredible.

Key Barriers and Indicators

The principal scientific concern relates to disease transmission between animals and humans. The pig is known to harbor a retrovirus, but there is no known transmission of any infection or disease from pigs to humans. In theory, any infectious agent could be bred out of the donor animal, but the threat of disease cannot be dismissed entirely, nor can the successful treatment of a transmitted infection be assured. Preliminary vaccination of the organ recipient is a feasible option that could confer additional protection. Another concern is excessive inbreeding, and one goal of creating herds of pig donors is to use as little inbreeding as possible.

Two issues will need to be addressed: the economic consequences of applying a new technology on a scale that today would seem to be vast but which is not precisely predictable, and the ethical and public policy implications of resource allocation and equity.

Wild Cards

- Managed care organizations develop the analytical tools to make rational trade-offs among different therapeutic modalities. Because of their cost-effectiveness, drug therapies offset a large share of medical costs. Drug spending as a share of total health spending increases from 9 percent to 20 percent. Meanwhile, overall health expenditures decline.

- Drug-resistant strains of staphylococcus and tuberculosis become commonplace, not just in developing countries but also in more affluent parts of the world's population. This spurs a renaissance in antibiotics research, but not before millions of lives are lost.

- Image-guided surgery from remote locations—telesurgery—becomes a common practice mode for procedures such as laparoscopies and chalecystectomies. Global centers of excellence develop for those procedures, driving many local specialists out of business.

ENDNOTES

[1] Ronchi, E. Biotechnology and the new revolution in health care and pharmaceuticals. Special Issue on biotechnology. *Science Technology Industry Review* 1996; 19:19–44.

[2] Jenks, S. J. Gene therapy: mastering the basics, defining details. *Journal of National Cancer Institute* 1997; 89,16:1182–84.

[3] Moxon, E. R. Applications of molecular microbiology to vaccinology. *Lancet* 1997; 350:1240–44.

CHAPTER 8

Information Technologies

Will Health Care Join in the Information Age?

Over the next decade, health care in the United States will at last be dramatically affected by the revolution in communications and information technology that has been in process for the past 15 years. Most information technologies, which have become a familiar part of the business landscape, are outgrowths of the increased power and reduced costs of microprocessors and lasers and the consequent cost reduction in both data processing and computer memory. Indeed, most businesses in the United States are now filled with networked personal computer (PC)

technologies (see Figures 8-1 and 8-2) that have migrated into households within the past 5 years (see Figure 8-3).

Although health care industry spending on information technology is projected to be as much as $21 billion in 2000,[1] health care has lagged behind other industries in adopting technology-enabled processes and has not experienced the dramatic changes in practices seen in finance, retail, distribution, and other industries. No health care company has used technology to change the way of

Figure 8-1. More and More PC Usage by the Workforce
(Percentage of workforce using personal computers)

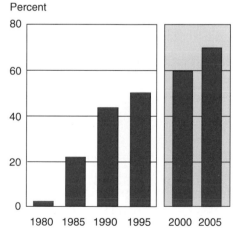

Source: IFTF; U.S. Bureau of Labor Statistics.

Figure 8-2. Percentage of PCs Connected to Local Area Networks (LANs)

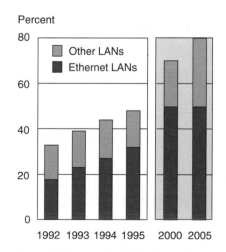

Source: IFTF; International Data Corporation.

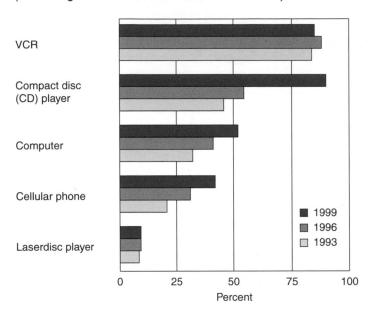

Figure 8-3. Technologies in the Home Take Off
(Percentage of United States households with . . .)

VCR

Compact disc
(CD) player

Computer

Cellular phone

Laserdisc player

■ 1999
■ 1996
□ 1993

0   25   50   75   100
Percent

Source: IFTF; Louis Harris & Associates, Television Bureau of Advertising, Recording Industry Association of America, International Recording Media Association.

There are two key fundamentals. The first is to understand the underlying cutting-edge technologies that will emerge from other industries and that will enjoy mass diffusion by 2010. The second is to understand which aspects of health care will be most affected by these technologies.

BASE TECHNOLOGIES

All of the applications and new processes that will change health care's use of information depend on developments in base technologies. The most important underlying technologies are listed below, with brief explanations of what they do now and what developments are likely.

■ *Microprocessors.* A microprocessor is the "brain" within computers that executes their functions. Moore's Law suggests that, as has been true for 30 years, microprocessors will continue to double in power every 18 to 24 months. This means that by the end of the next decade, PCs will have a processing capacity some 30 times faster than they have today, and powerful processors will be found in virtually every manufactured product, including clothes, furniture, and buildings, as well as cars and consumer electronics. Medical devices and information systems will also benefit from increased processing power.

■ *Data storage.* Enabled by the development, in the late 1980s, of cheap lasers—the key to both compact discs and large-capacity optical storage systems—data storage capacity has fallen in price to the point where technology planners believe that it will soon be

doing business as dramatically as Wal-Mart changed retailing, for instance, or Charles Schwab transformed securities brokering. But it's clear that changes in information technology will continue to be one of, if not *the,* prime catalyst of health care change over the next 10 years. Can we then expect a shift toward the prevalence of automated customer service, electronic information exchange, and real-time data analysis that's commonplace in those other industries? As health care tries to assimilate currently available technologies, new types of, and uses for, information technology are emerging at a rapid and increasing pace. How will health care adapt to incorporating a host of new technologies over the next decade?

nearly free. Consequently very large data sets, such as entire film outputs from years of MRI use, can be captured and stored. Those files are then accessible for searching, processing, and analyzing.

■ *Software tools.* Software is the instruction that enables processors to perform their tasks. Programming software has been a specialized operation, but increasingly the tools to create software are simpler and more fault resistant. The ease with which World Wide Web pages can now be created by amateurs, where just 5 years ago it took training in computer programming just to use the Internet, is an example of this shift. In the future, object-oriented software potentially will eliminate the need to write code, allowing computer operators to change applications.

■ *Networking and data compression.* Networks that permit information transfer among computers have exploded in prevalence and utility. With higher-bandwidth networks and with new techniques in compressing data so that more information can be saved in the same amount of computer storage, larger amounts of data will be transferred at higher speeds among more users. Health care providers, especially radiologists and others working together on large-image files, will benefit from this trend.

■ *Information appliances.* The most common information appliance is the computer, but increasingly the components and functions of computers will appear in telephones, televisions,

and other devices. The class and number of information appliances will accelerate dramatically.

■ *Intelligent agents.* Software programs that find and retrieve information over a network that is likely to be helpful to an end user, even though the user doesn't know where that information is coming from, will grow in popularity. Current intelligent agents are somewhat crude, but over the next few years their filtering and retrieval ability will increase dramatically.

■ *Security and encryption.* The transmission of medical and financial information will depend on the full distribution of encryption technologies that permit secure transmission of data. The underlying technology for encryption is developing fast, but the procedures ensuring that all transmissions are secure will be difficult to implement.

■ *Internet and the World Wide Web.* Although the Internet as we know it will scarcely be recognizable in a decade's time, its current incarnation provides a common format for viewing, exchanging, and transacting information of all kinds that is transferable among different computer systems. In particular, the volume of transactions conducted over the Internet—as opposed to the simple one-way sharing of information—will increase dramatically.

■ *3-D computing.* Data visualization is the use of computing to represent huge volumes of data in three dimensions on one computer screen. The

Chapter 8: Information Technologies   **111**

ability to move, shape, and analyze data in ways that support decision making will enable managers to view activities, classes of transactions, and entire organizations in whole and in detail at the same time.

- *Databases.* A new class of both relational and object-oriented databases will increase the capacity to store, present, sort, and analyze data over the next decade. Even though these new database systems will be incompatible with older "legacy" databases, a considerable amount of older information will be extracted from those databases by using techniques called "data warehousing" and "data mining."

- *Sensors.* The real world can connect with computers by using devices such as digital video cameras or blood pressure monitors. A key change of the next decade will be the fall in the cost of sensors, making sensors an integral part of many computing devices and information appliances. Their great diffusion will allow the monitoring of events that previously went unreported or were very costly to track.

- *Expert systems.* Computer applications programmed with a set of rules that codify experts' assessments of particular situations are known as expert systems. The combination of that technology with informational inputs allows these systems to suggest options and outcome probabilities. They can support humans making all kinds of decisions, including those governing medical care.

Given the progress made so far and the massive international commercial investment in information technology research and development, we can expect continued rapid advances in and diffusion of these basic technologies over the next decade. For health care, which has been behind the curve, both the application of currently available information technologies and the development of new technologies will combine to cause dramatic change.

THE ISSUES: THE DIRECTION IS CLEAR, THE PACE UNCERTAIN

While it's possible to imagine some incredible impacts of information technology on health care, the implementation of new information systems is a task barely begun. There are all kinds of organizational, financial, and educational barriers preventing adoption of different technologies and all kinds of difficulties with their use when they are adopted. Several major information system ventures in health care have failed, particularly clinical information systems. The planned exchange of information over dedicated local networks (like the Community Health Information Networks of the early 1990s) also went nowhere despite much effort. The next decade will see much greater change than in the last. But we need to be clear about what we're projecting.

Information systems in health care are used for administrative, clinical, and financial purposes. Most systems have elements of all three activities, but administrative and financial transactions are already much more automated than most clinical ones. For example, about half of all claims are sent electronically, whereas well under 5 percent of physicians use computers to record all clinical information for an average patient. A similar difference exists among hospitals using computer systems to automate their admission and registration functions but paper charts to record nursing activities. The adoption of electronic transactions varies dramatically by sector for the same type of transaction, with physicians' offices typically being the least automated (see Figure 8-4).

Given that information systems will be used to convert health care from paper to electronic recording—but at a different rate depending on the activity and organization—there are some key questions: How fast will different types of technologies diffuse? What kinds of organizations will use what types of technologies and for what purposes? Who will pay for them and who will benefit? While there will be no part of the health care system that doesn't see change caused or enabled by information technology, we believe that four major areas will see the greatest impact.

THE FORECAST: FOUR BIG EFFECTS IN HEALTH CARE

Although health care will use information technology in a variety of ways, we think the most important effects will be in four main areas:

- process-management systems
- clinical information interfaces
- data analysis
- telehealth and remote monitoring

PROCESS-MANAGEMENT SYSTEMS

Provider and Plan Management Systems Go Electronic

The first major area where information technology will affect health care is in the automation of basic business processes among providers and intermediaries and their customers. These processes include provider network contract administration, communications between different organizations over administrative issues, such as patient eligibility and claims submission, and the business and medical protocols used in customer service centers. These developments occupy the broad category of "electronic commerce."

Figure 8-4. Electronic Health Care Claims Pick Up the Pace (Percentage of electronic claims by source)

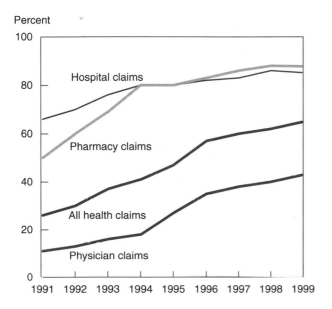

Source: Faulkner and Gray.

Electronic commerce is being encouraged by cheaper and more flexible technologies, such as transactions conducted over the Internet and other open and cheaply accessible computer networks. But the major driving force behind the adoption of electronic commerce in health care is the combination of mandated standards for electronic data exchange and the regulatory incentives to use them legislated in the 1996 Kennedy–Kassebaum Act (officially known as HIPAA). While the low-hanging fruit of insurance and administrative simplification standards have seen final rules published, several areas have been controversial and have not yet been finalized. Consensus has been impossible in the area of privacy, and particularly in regard to the National Individual Identifier for patients. Congress failed to enact legislation governing such standards by August 21, 1999. The deadline for the Secretary of Health and Human Services to publish the final standards for privacy of individually identifiable health information is February 21, 2000.

We can expect several prominent functions to be performed electronically by the early years of the next decade. These include claims submission, eligibility verification, coordination of insurance benefits between providers, utilization review and precertification, materials management, pharmacy claims, and utilization review and receipt of lab tests. So the technology-enabled processes that manage the everyday interactions of health plans, providers, and patients will change dramatically—and quite soon.

These administrative links between providers and plans will be comple-

mented by better use of computing and telephony links among plans or providers and their members and payers, including employers. Telephone-based customer service centers with human staffs are likely to remain the largest single example of this interaction, but other links will be emblematic of this convergence of technology and process. These include automated enrollment by using interactive voice response (IVR) or the Internet, administrative information and health information delivered by a combination of phone, mail, and computer, and even the development of online insurance markets. These secondary electronic commerce developments will become mainstream after 2005.

CLINICAL INFORMATION INTERFACES

The EMR has been an elusive promise of technology for at least a decade.[2] The concept is that all medical information about a patient should be stored electronically to be accessed whenever, wherever, and by whomever needs it, and that data need be input only once. That system would loop information back from the patient to the physician, pharmacist, and case manager, permitting medical management in real time rather than retrospectively. This ideal would require ubiquitous use of information technology. But as Figure 8-5 shows, by 1997—more than 10 years into the PC revolution—few physicians used computers in their everyday clinical practice.

Nonetheless, many of the components that would support an EMR, such as databases, networks, and computers, are being put into place. Furthermore, the past few years have seen the development of sophisticated software tools that support clinical practice. What has been missing to jumpstart the EMR is an easily usable interface that helps clinicians get information into and out of computer systems as fast as they can write on paper, or that at least gives them a payoff for investing in the system's use.

Over the next decade, ubiquitous information appliances, sophisticated decision support systems, and voice recognition will create interfaces with computing systems that are much more clinician-friendly. Consequently, we're likely to see more input of clinical observations into electronic databases and more information being fed back from these systems to clinicians at the point of care. The clinicians' interface will link to most areas of health information systems but will follow a close codevelopment

with aspects of clinical databases and analytical tools. So we will be moving closer, incrementally, to an EMR.

The rate of change toward prevalent use of the EMR will depend on the economics driving the adoption of these systems, which currently can cost up to $50,000 per clinician. While the price of the systems will fall, most of the cost actually resides in the implementation and education that is required. Currently the initial training alone is estimated to be at least 48 hours per physician.[3] Of course there are advantages to using EMRs that are also measurable in cost terms, including faster access to data, lower rates of retesting as is required when original results can't be found, and often more accurate care as in the case of fewer adverse drug reactions.[4]

Both the increased importance of non-physician clinicians and the fact that younger physicians have greater experience with computers will drive this increased use of clinical information technology. Many health care organizations are also developing into an economic size and type that gives them the financial and management resources to automate clinical activities. Many organizations have announced plans to implement clinical information systems for clinician use. Their reasons stem partly from pressure from intermediaries and end payers for better reporting and partly from a belief that improving the clinical process will give them a competitive advantage in the future. The economic value of automating the clinical process will drive its adoption particularly in payment environments that reward lower costs, such as capitation.

Figure 8-5. Which Clinical Functions Do Physicians Perform with Computers?

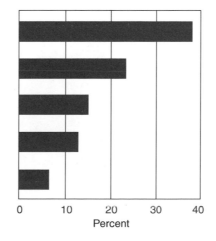

Access background information, such as Medline, via Internet or online service

Access clinical patient information

Record patients' clinical information, such as histories

Transmit clinical information to other doctors electronically

Receive computerized treatment protocols

Percent

Source: Health Care Outlook Physicians Survey, 1997; Healtheon; Louis Harris & Associates.

In order to encourage physicians to use this technology, more effort will focus on finding ways to educate and encourage physicians to change their behavior. The pursuit of that goal will lead to greater study of the clinical decision-making process as a whole and the best way to use information technology to influence decisions at the time they are made.

However, the dissemination of clinical information systems into the daily practice of clinicians will be a slow process. Clinicians will start to use computers more as part of their regular work, including accessing and recording patient information, usually in a hybrid paper/computer approach. But the ideal of the EMR will not come about easily. A number of other information systems challenges, such as the Year 2000 problem, a lack of capital, and continued resistance from clinicians, will mean that only a small percentage of physicians and clinicians will be conducting their practice using fully computerized medical records until later in the next decade.

Within the move toward information systems that clinicians can integrate into their daily work, two models are developing for the future EMR. One will focus on giving clinicians access to clinical information, such as lab results, transcripts, and demographic data, that is currently already available over information networks. These systems will accept physicians' input in any way they can, including voice, handwriting scans, and free text. These systems will concentrate on presenting as much relevant data to the clinician as possible and getting this implementation widespread quickly.

The other approach will also try to provide these data but will go the extra mile to have physicians input their notes in a structured format, either using check boxes or menus or allowing them to type. The system will then use natural language processing technology to codify and assign values to their words. The idea is to capture and analyze physicians' clinical assessments of patients, as that's where the most valuable information resides. The codifying of that clinical assessment will permit better analysis for outcomes studies, provider profiling, and eventually for assessing the value of interventions in close to real time—potentially changing the model of how information about clinical practice is disseminated. This model demands far more involvement from clinicians and more resources from their organizations and will probably diffuse more slowly. After the next decade, these EMRs may include expert systems that support clinicians' decision making and incorporate many of the analytical tools now being developed on the database side discussed below.

DATA ANALYSIS

The analysis of health care data is a growth industry. In the next few years, more data will be collected from diverse input sources, including clinicians, patients, other clinical data sources, and administrative and claims data systems. We are already seeing improvements in the use of databases and data warehouses to store and link disparate data streams; likewise, the ability of analysts to visualize and deconstruct complex data sets is improving. Both data mining and database design will improve dramatically in the coming decade, but the most important aspect of this technology will be sophisticated data manipulation. Two related trends in data manipulation are likely to emerge from this core technology, both involving attempts to better understand the impact of clinical interventions and in particular how clinical interventions affect outcomes.

In the shorter term, a great deal of effort will be aimed at pulling clinical information from what are largely administrative data sets. A new group of sophisticated "data jockeys" will give plans and providers the tools to learn much more about patients' clinical outcomes from particular interventions. This trend will lead to:

■ Better decision-making support for internal and competitive analysis, which will be aided by improved computing that permits 3-D visualization of complex data sets.

■ Better understanding of patients' likelihood of future illness.

■ The ability to adjust payments to plans depending on the relative risk of illness of an enrolled population. This "risk adjustment" will be based in part on a much wider use of patients' self-assessment to understand their own health status.

Medicare will start to use risk-adjustment algorithms to change the amount it reimburses health plans after 2000, at which point the importance of data analysis will increase. Clinicians attempting to understand the costs of care for their patients with different acuity levels won't merely be seeing theoretical sav-

ings down the road but instead will have to manage the care they deliver in order to receive those savings. Data mining is already being used by retail companies, computer marketers, and professional basketball teams—we expect dramatic growth in this type of analysis in medical care by the year 2002.

In the longer term, more codified and analyzable clinical data will be available directly recorded from the clinician–patient interface. The data will probably include patients' genetic information and not only will provide greater understanding about patients' experiences and outcomes but also will better monitor the performance of both clinicians and patients. The emergence of online analytical processing will permit close to real-time analysis of the key information, such as the result of a particular intervention. This is in contrast to the retrospective analysis that's done today, and will be an addition to, and an improvement on, the analysis based on data mining of administrative data sets described in the previous paragraph. However, analytical processing of clinical data will not be more than a fringe activity until a majority of clinicians are using EMRs. That will take several years and won't be prevalent until well after 2005.

Some of this data analysis will be made publicly available through regulatory agencies and bodies like the NCQA, which accredits health plans. Consequently, the ability of more organizations and individuals to access information about the type and quality of care provided will increase later in the next decade.

Telehealth and Remote Monitoring

Combining Case Management, Patient Information Systems, and Remote Monitoring

In the long term, the impact of all these technologies will be greatest on patient care. There are three main trends that will converge in their use of interconnecting technologies to provide remote care. The trends are case management, patient information systems, and remote telemetry.

Case Management Gets Automated

Plans and providers will use automated techniques to case manage patients. Most use of case management will concentrate on the process of disease state or chronic care management. Disease management organizations, whether providers or intermediaries, will use protocols, clinical information, software, and infrastructure that have been developed to support that process. The protocols will make use of mathematical models that assess appropriate treatment for specific conditions and data collected on individual patients. The data will be manipulated both to improve the treatment options of the individual patients and to add to larger databases. Case managers will use medical records and protocols to track and assess treatment patterns, and the growth of call centers will help deliver that information to patients.

Empowered Patients Get Informed

Some of the same technologies that providers will use for medical management will also have an impact on patients independently. Patients will use them for a variety of health information activities that will include shared decision making, psychosocial support groups, disease-specific information research, physician and provider assessment, information about alternative medicine, and patient self-care support tools, such as software that tracks diet and treatment regimens. Empowerment of patients via information gathering will center on use of the Internet and other online services, IVR, CD-ROMs, video, and television, including video-on-demand over cable and satellite networks.

Most of the activity already happening in this area has been inspired by patients and is somewhat anarchic in nature. That won't change any time soon, but there will be significant entry of plans, providers, and other actors into this arena who will try to impose a more structured use of information sources so that they can guide and track the treatment of their patients.

One problem we foresee is that the chronically ill and elderly tend not to have the necessary technology in their homes. Figure 8-6 shows that while 50 percent of American households had computers in 1998, computers were much more likely to be in households with higher income, better education, younger age, and better health status. By the year 2003, 63 percent of American households will have appliances with processing power equivalent to a PC, increasing to 65 to 70 percent by 2006 (see Figure 8-7). There's also a significant possibility that America's information have-nots will not get access to the ser-

Figure 8-6. Technology in Households Is Mostly for the Wealthy and Educated (Percentage of U.S. households with PCs, by education and income, 1998)

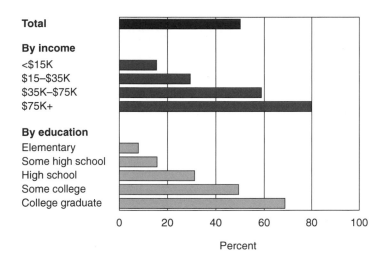

Source: IFTF; National Telecommunications and Information Administration.

Figure 8-7. Internet and Computer Penetration of the Household Will Continue to Increase (Percentage of U.S. households with PCs and Internet connections)

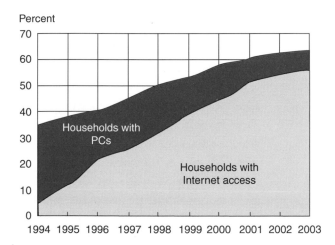

Source: Forrester Research, 1999.

vices associated with these technologies. Surveys of Internet use[5] taken in 1998 show that fewer than 10 percent of Internet users were age 55 years or older (21 percent of Americans are in that age category). Further, in 1998, 26 percent of Americans over 55 had home computers, but only 14 percent of those over 55 had accessed online services.

Access to information technology will be an area of public policy contention in the next few years, and possibly of some marker activity as manufacturers get the capacity to introduce Internet-like services in lower-cost devices, such as network computers, game machines, and TVs, and as these become affordable for everyone. If these appliances can be used for accessing online information, there's no reason to believe that they won't be nearly as common as color TV, with more than 95 percent of households having the processing and communications power of a current top-end PC soon after 2005.

Sensors Boost Remote Telemetry

The final piece of the puzzle needed for remote care to really take off is the monitoring function that connects the case managers to the patients. While education and self-care are necessary components that will be facilitated by information technology, clinical assessment of patients has to this point required that they either be at a medical facility or be attended to in their own homes by expensive labor, But a new type of technology is becoming available that will set off a revolution in remote care because it will provide the capacity for remote telemetry. The technology is the sensor, which converts analog, or real-life, signals into digital format, which computer systems can understand and therefore report on and react to.

The sensors that are being created for automobiles, video cameras, and all manner of other electronics will become cheap enough to drive their adoption in medical devices. Examples of how sensors may be used in remote telemetry include monitoring vital signs with wireless heart monitors; integrating digital signal creation by wireless or intermittently wired monitors, such as respiratory meters, blood pressure cuffs, or blood glucose monitors, with patient, plan, or provider information systems; and providing alerts from pharmaceutical dispensers that a needed pill hasn't been taken. At the back end of all these devices will be a link into the software for disease management or provider information organizations that will analyze, report, and react to abnormal results or the absence of them. This, in turn, should ensure appropriate follow-up, for instance a visit from a nurse, in more cases and better use of resources.

Inventing new ways of getting these technologies and the networks that support them into homes and smaller medical facilities will be an area of focus over the next 10 years, and these new approaches will draw on the experience of other industries, notably entertainment. In addition to monitoring the chronically ill, who tend to be high-end resource users, similar technologies will be used for patients' self-monitoring, including results reporting using a phone or computer—typically for those with less severe chronic conditions. For

instance, lab testing will become increasingly decentralized. Advances in self-diagnosis with small, portable testing devices and immune assays will also be increasingly important. An example might be the "smart toilet," a very simple-to-use device that tests for problems in the digestive system. Results from these devices will be captured in computer systems and monitored in a similar way to the more active telemetry.

PROGRESSION OF INFORMATION TECHNOLOGY INTO HEALTH CARE

The four areas we've defined—process-management systems, clinical information interfaces, data analysis, and remote monitoring—are not the only aspects of information technology that will have an impact on health care,[6] although they are dominant themes that will encapsulate a great deal of the change that information technology will bring to health care. But it will not be an equal progression. The advent of electronic commerce will transform administrative processes in the next few years, and the new ways of administration will be ubiquitous by 2007. While great strides will have been made in other areas, the use of information systems by clinicians as an integral part of their work—the key vision of the EMR—will only develop in the latter part of the next decade and will not be complete by 2010. However, the use of information systems will change the roles of the patient and the case manager intermediary in the next 10 years. Patients will become more informed and involved in their own care plans, and intermediaries responsible for medical management will use information technology extensively to assess cases in real time. Physicians will adapt their practice to adjust to this, but at a slow pace.

The adoption of technology will depend on the ability of health care organizations to set aside capital for investment and therefore depends on the ability of those organizations to become more like other types of corporations. While health care is moving in this direction (e.g., growth of physician groups), it will remain a fragmented industry that, as it consolidates, will struggle with the adoption and deployment of information technology. The use of that technology as an enabling driver to change health care will not really be felt until those consolidated organizations are more stable, after 2005. By that time, the cost of the more complex clinical information systems will have fallen to the point that its widespread adoption need not be put off for economic reasons. After that, the vision of an information-intensive industry using information technology for consumer-friendly, high-quality, and low-cost patient care can become a real possibility.

WILD CARDS

- With a new generation of software and hardware, diffusion of clinical information technology happens fully in the next 3 to 5 years. The EMR becomes commonplace, patients' records are standardized, and the clinical care process dramatically improves.

- Federal legislation on privacy of patient information stops the ability of health care organizations to electronically share health information. The development of EMRs and even the exchange of administrative information with clinical components starts to fade.

- Early large-scale implementation of information systems to support and case manage the chronically ill show no cost-benefit advantages compared to traditional lower-end technology care. Given the cost of system installation, the development of home monitoring and case management remains in its current embryonic state.

- The Year 2000 problem creates a major systems crisis with more serious consequences than had been anticipated and spreads to almost all equipment in health care. Through 2001, almost all staffing resources have to be redeployed to sort out current systems, delaying all other advances in information technology to much later in the decade.

- The spread of information technology to consumers is very rapid. By 2005 all patients have access to as much information as medical professionals. Substantial numbers of these informed patients reject physicians and plans and become their own care managers. Alternate care providers, physicians, pharmacists, and facilities all lose their professional status and become commodities as consumers use them as undifferentiated suppliers.

ENDNOTES

[1] Sheldon Dorenfest & Co.

[2] In its 1991 report, *The Computer-Based Patient Record,* the Institute of Medicine listed areas of technology that, when integrated, would make up a computer-based patient record (CPR). The technologies included databases and database management systems, workstations, data acquisition and retrieval, image processing and storage, data exchange and vocabulary standards, and system communications and network infrastructure.

[3] See Krall, M. A. Acceptance and performance by clinicians using an ambulatory electronic medical record in an HMO. *Proceedings of Annual Symposium of Computer Applications in Medical Care* 1995; 708–11 for a generally positive description of the implementation of the Epic EMR at Kaiser Northwest.

[4] See Bares, D. W., et al. Incidence of adverse drug events and potential adverse drug events: implications for prevention. *Journal of the American Medical Association* (July 5) 1995; 274(1):29–34. This describes the problems with drug interactions and other mistakes that Brigham and Womens Hospital more or less eliminated by switching to a computerized ordering system. See also Anderson, J. G., et al. Evaluating the potential effectiveness of using computerized information systems to prevent adverse drug events. *Proceedings of AMIA Annual Fall Symposium* 1997; 9:228–32.

[5] *Falling Through the Net: Defining the Digital Divide.* Washington, DC: National Telecommunications and Information Administration, July 1999.

[6] For instance, telemedicine today is a fringe activity in which physician consults occur over dedicated videoconferencing facilities. This will stay a fringe activity, but some telemedicine will transmute into the use of groupware (computer communications) to share information between care teams and the use of online environments for collaboration between clinicians. In another example, the production of digital signals from imaging equipment will dramatically increase radiologists' ability to use computers to analyze and abstract information from X rays, MR images, and other imaging devices.

CHAPTER 9

Health Care Consumers

The Haves and the Have-Nots

We define "health care consumer" as anyone who receives or has the potential to receive health care services, regardless of whether or not that person pays for those services directly. Although employers and government, not health care consumers, are the most frequent purchasers of health insurance and thus pay for a great deal of the care provided, we discuss them in this chapter only in the context of their effects on individual consumers.

Consumers are more actively engaged in their own health care than in the past. Up until the mid-1980s, health care consumers in the United States generally had been passive recipients of care. Most patients submitted to whatever procedures a physician recommended, and most were happy to let the system take responsibility for decisions about their care. By and large, mainstream Americans revered doctors and trusted them— a culture sustained by the large information gap between highly educated doctors and the average patient. It was a gap further reinforced by doctors' political and economic power.

Patients' impact on the organization of care was also slight because employers and government, not patients, were—as they still are—the purchasers of health

care for a majority of working adults. Employers typically offered little choice among health insurance plans to their employees, making it difficult for patients to vote with their feet if they were dissatisfied with their coverage. Yet because traditional indemnity plans allowed free choice of provider, and because employers and government generally provided health care coverage as a defined benefit with low out-of-pocket costs, consumers' lack of plan choice did not seem to affect their care or their pocketbooks much, keeping dissatisfaction low among insured consumers. The uninsured have made do with limited coverage from safety-net funding streams and providers—a mix of public institutions and private charity—and have not had many advocates to speak for them. Although insured consumers and their advocates have had some impact on insurance legislation over the years, they have had little impact on the delivery of care. Their legislative voice has been muted in part because they haven't had many big issues to complain about.

As a consequence of these three factors— a culture of respect for physicians and their power sustained by an information gap, employer- and government-mediated purchasing, and defined benefits with free choice of providers—consumers have had relatively little effect on the organization of American health care. Until recently, providers (mostly hospitals and physicians in solo practice or small-group practice), health care plans, and purchasers (mostly employers and government) controlled how and where care was provided, who got it, and how much it cost the individual out-of-pocket in premiums, deductibles, and most recently, copayments. Individual consumers adapted to the system.

That picture is changing. As a new, more educated and informed generation of baby boomer consumers moves through the system and reaches the age where they use more health care services, a new culture of assertive skepticism is replacing the old culture of passivity and respect. A rapidly growing group of consumers is trusting plans and providers less, demanding more information and choice from providers and plans, engaging in more self-care and self-management of disease, and showing more interest in sharing their health care decisions with providers. Choice, self-care, and shared decision making are the key elements of consumer empowerment covered by our forecast.

As baby boomers reach an age where they require doctor visits more frequently, employers are beginning to pass more health care costs on to employees, often by replacing defined benefits programs with defined contribution programs—thus potentially weakening employer mediation of consumption. The managed care revolution, triggered by escalating national health care costs has limited consumers' choice of providers and forced them to negotiate a thicket of primary care gatekeepers, access charges for specialists, and triage nurses on telephones in order to get the care they need. Combined with rising out-of-pocket costs, these limits have given the new, more informed and vocal consumers something to complain about. Change in the consumers' role is definitely in the wind.

The Three Modes of Empowerment

Informed Choice of Plans and Providers: The combination of employers' shifting to defined contribution programs and the increasing openness of provider networks available through plans will lead to a greater range of choices of providers and plans. Consumers will demand more sophisticated and comparative information about plans and providers to help them make these choices.

Self-Care and Self-Management: Increasing consumer access to medical information formerly known only to providers, combined with improved remote sensing technologies, will facilitate greater involvement of patients in their own health care, including preventive care (e.g., improving diet and lifestyle), treating acute episodes at home, and helping manage the course of their chronic diseases.

Shared Medical Decision Making: Improved medical record systems and increasingly sophisticated decision-support tools will facilitate patients' ability to understand complex medical decision-making processes and become more active in choosing treatments that match their preferences and values.

Will the historically supply-driven health care market soon be forced to grapple with consumer demands? Will such changes be large and noticeable by 2010, or only incremental? To answer these questions, we need to know which consumers are likely to drive change the most, what changes they are likely to push most quickly, what forces will resist them, and what impact the changes are likely to have on providers, purchasers,

The Aging Baby Boomers

Baby boomers make up the generation born between 1945 and 1964. The first baby boomers will turn 65 in 2010. The percentage of the population that is over age 65 has been steadily increasing in this century, but the baby boomers will drive that percentage sharply higher (see figure 9-1). Over the next 15 years, the baby boom cohort will move into its 50s and will begin to experience more chronic and severe illnesses. Those who are "new consumers" will be a particularly strong voice for change.

Figure 9-1. Population Age 65 and Older, 1980 to 2030

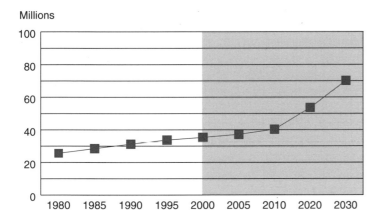

Source: U.S. Census Bureau, Statistical Abstract, 1996.

and plans. Will the overall impact on the system within the coming decade be striking, or a yawn?

To get at the answer, we first identify the three tiers of coverage into which consumers currently fall and the key issues facing each tier. We then forecast the changes most likely to occur in each tier and their implications for the system. We also take a look at some wild cards and identify a few emerging consumer needs that health care services may be able to fill in the future.

THREE TIERS OF HEALTH CARE CONSUMERS

Although legislators frequently hold up the ideal of a one-tier health care system, plans requiring major redistribution of resources have not been well received in Congress or by the public. In reality, three tiers exist.

The bottom tier is the rapidly growing group of Americans who lack access to the main system and are served largely by an increasingly tattered safety net because they are either uninsured or on Medicaid; currently, the number of uninsured is about 42 million when measured at a single point in time and about one-quarter of those are children.

The middle tier consists of those working Americans whose benefits are insecure because of threats to their jobs due to restructuring or ailing industries, low reemployability, employer benefits cuts, restrictions on providers and treatments, or potential inability to pay the insurance premiums passed on to them by their employers.

The top tier is made up of the very wealthy and the more securely employed, who have fewer restrictions on their care. The current system thus consists of a disenfranchised bottom tier (the excluded consumer), an insecurely enfranchised middle tier (the worried consumer), and a securely enfranchised top tier (the empowered consumer).

An alternative way to define the three tiers would be by the continuity of their insurance—to look at who is continu-

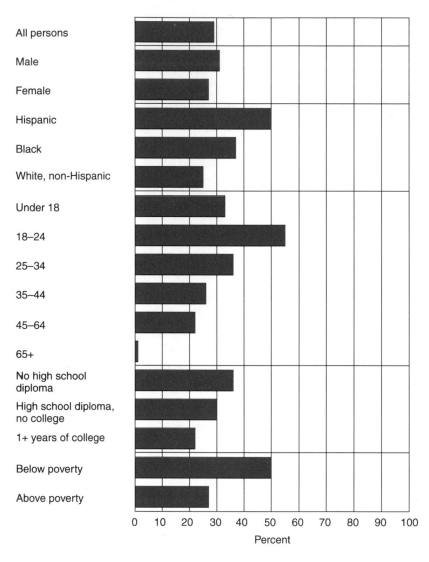

Figure 9-2. Benefits Insecurity

	0	10	20	30	40	50	60	70	80	90	100
All persons											
Male											
Female											
Hispanic											
Black											
White, non-Hispanic											
Under 18											
18–24											
25–34											
35–44											
45–64											
65+											
No high school diploma											
High school diploma, no college											
1+ years of college											
Below poverty											
Above poverty											

Percent

Source: U.S. Census Bureau.

ously insured, insured on and off, and continuously uninsured during a given period. If we examine the years between 1993 and 1996, we find that about 71 percent of Americans were continuously insured, 25 percent lacked coverage between 1 and 35 months, and 4 percent were continuously uninsured (see Figure 9-2). These three groups were further divided along ethnic lines: 50 percent of Hispanics lacked coverage for a month or more as compared to 37 percent of African Americans and 25 percent of whites.

The problem with using continuity of coverage as a means of defining the tiers is that many who are continuously insured are nonetheless worried about either the stability or the flexibility of their benefits. Furthermore, some of the insured have only very limited coverage, including those on Medicaid.

For those reasons, we have chosen to define the three tiers by the degree to which their benefits are adequate and perceived to be secure. Although we recognize that a fair amount of movement goes on between tiers, the three tiers themselves persist.

The consumers most likely to become empowered in the coming decade are the "new consumers" (see Figure 9-2). In contrast to traditional consumers, new consumers have at least two of the following three attributes: at least 1 year of college education, more than $50,000 in household income, and experience with information technology (e.g., computers). Because education, income, and experience with information technology are closely linked, most of the disenfranchised bottom tier consists of traditional consumers. Significant segments of the middle and upper tiers, however, are new consumers, including a large proportion of the baby boom generation.

Chapter 9: Health Care Consumers

The New Consumers: Who Are They?

We define new consumers as people who have at least two of the following three characteristics:

1. Discretionary household income of $53,000 or more (in constant 1998 dollars)
2. At least 1 year of college education
3. Experience with information technology (e.g., owns a PC)

Figure 9-3. Description of New Consumer Attributes in 2005 (Percentage of group without health insurance for at least 1 month out of 36 months, 1993 to 1996)

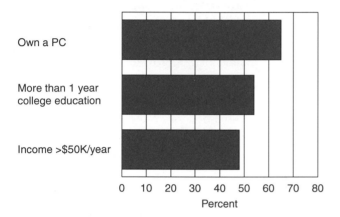

Source: IFTF; U.S. Department of Labor.

In other sectors of the economy, such as retail and banking, the new consumers have already initiated a revolution in the way goods are purchased and customers are served. These consumers are also narrowing the patient–provider information gap. They are no longer in awe of physicians, and they will be the first to demand change from health care plans and providers as they interact with the system between now and 2010. In discussing the key issues facing each tier, we highlight the points at which the new consumers may have the most impact.

THE BOTTOM TIER: THE DISENFRANCHISED AND NEVER-ENFRANCHISED

The main issue for the disenfranchised, of course, is access to health care.[1] This tier consists of people under 65 who are uninsured, including a significant number of children, or who have very limited insurance—mostly through Medicaid, and a very small number on both Medicare and Medicaid. In 1998, 5 percent of the population in the United States comprised adults covered by Medicaid, 12 percent were uninsured adults, 5 percent were children on Medicaid, and 4 percent were uninsured children, for a total of 26 percent of the population in the bottom tier.

Access to care for this tier is severely limited because the safety net has become frayed . People in this tier depend utterly on the limited resources and strained generosity of safety-net funding streams and providers. Even those on Medicaid have limited choices. A significant proportion of people on Medicaid are mothers and children receiving AFDC. Their benefits depend on state budgets, where they compete for resources with prisons and schools.

Recent welfare reform bills have limited eligibility for Medicaid, particularly where immigrants are concerned. In a 1995 survey of state officials, 65 percent thought that in the next 3 years their state was likely to place tighter constraints on care for Medicaid patients than it permitted for privately insured patients.

Children: Patients and Beneficiaries, but Not Active Consumers

In 1998, children under age 18 made up roughly 27 percent of the United States population. Roughly one-third of this group, representing 9 percent of the total population, lacked coverage for at least 1 month in a 36-month period between 1993 and 1996.

Although we include children in our estimates of the percentage of the population falling into each tier—and the problem of uninsured children is a serious one—we do not discuss them further in this section because they are generally not active purchasers of or participants in their health care and will therefore exert little influence over it.

Generally poor and lacking a college education, most people in the bottom tier will have serious trouble overcoming the information gap between providers and patients. Even the new consumers in this tier, the not-yet-insured recent college graduates who have not yet found stable jobs, will have trouble—but most quickly move up to the middle and top tiers.

THE MIDDLE TIER: THE INSECURELY ENFRANCHISED

The primary issue for the middle tier is benefits security. When unemployment is high, this tier is insecure about maintaining coverage. When unemployment is low, they are insecure about maintaining the flexibility and quality of coverage. Although at any one time most of this tier is insured, their benefits are not secure for a variety of reasons. Adults in the middle tier include (1) working people with unstable job security, including employees and owners of small or downsizing businesses, contract employees, and employees of companies undergoing restructuring; and (2) early retirees (age 55 to 64 years) waiting for Medicare to kick in. We estimate that roughly 34

percent of the United States population falls into the middle tier.

The working group is worried because many of their employers are reducing or eliminating health care benefits or passing their costs on to employees, who may be unable to pay. Unstable job security and uncertain reemployability also put middle-tier members at risk for significant time periods without health insurance. The coverage this group does have tends increasingly to be in the form of HMO or PPO coverage, which limits to some extent both covered procedures and choice of providers.

Some early retirees are insecurely enfranchised because employers are increasingly cutting or restricting pension health benefits. Those benefits may include either managed care plans or traditional indemnity insurance. In 1997, 31 percent of employers offered health benefits to their Medicare-eligible retirees compared to 40 percent in 1993.

Closely related to benefits security is the issue of value. As employers cut their premium contributions and reduce the scope of the benefits they offer, costs are increasingly passed on to the consumers in this tier and value—the amount of coverage per dollar spent—becomes more of an issue.

The new consumer segment of this tier—which is growing rapidly—will be the most informed about their choices and the most likely to demand good information to help them make those choices, taking a step in the direction of empowerment. As independent agencies and, increasingly, health plans have begun to generate "report cards" for employers on plans and providers, the information-savvy new consumer segment may take advantage of them. As middle-tier members increasingly gain access to PCs at home and at work, the Internet will be a rapidly growing and easily accessible source of plan and provider information.

In contrast, most of the traditional consumers in this tier have at most a high school education and thus tend to have lower incomes and less exposure to information technology. The patient–provider information gap will be hard for this segment of the tier to overcome.

THE TOP TIER: THE SECURELY ENFRANCHISED

The primary issue for the securely enfranchised tier will be empowerment. Although the changes that this tier drives in the system will be slow and incremental at first, they have the greatest ability to effect change. This tier consists mainly of consumers who are (1) securely employed or highly employable, (2) very wealthy and often self-insured, or (3) elderly and on Medicare, either with or without supplemental private insurance.

Many members of this tier are employed by large companies, many of which offer plans with generous benefits designs, pay the lion's share if not all of premiums, and offer a choice of several different health insurance plans.

Medicare currently offers a rich benefits package, mostly FFS, although that is changing as Medicare HMOs become increasingly competitive.

Like the middle tier, the top tier consists of a mix of traditional and new consumers, with significant numbers in each category. Most of those over 65 in the top tier are traditional consumers. However, a large proportion of the group is made up of baby boomers who will turn 50 during the next decade. These new consumers will be interacting more and more with the system, and they will become a powerful force for change in the delivery of care.

People in the top tier are generally continuously insured in any given 2-year period. When they *do* lose their jobs, they are quickly reemployed thanks to their high level of education. In recent years, about 61 percent of the total United States population has been continuously insured by a plan other than Medicaid during any given 2-year period. Some are securely insured, some insecurely insured. About 13 percent of the population is covered by Medicare, usually supplemented by private insurance. We estimate that about 38 percent of the population constitute securely enfranchised consumers who thus fall into the top tier of coverage.

SUMMARY OF THE THREE TIERS

About one-third of the United States population currently falls into the middle tier of coverage, with a bit less than one-third occupying the bottom tier and a bit more than one-third the top tier (see Table 9-1). New consumers, who represent the largest potential for driving care delivery change in the next decade, are concentrated in the middle and upper tiers.

Table 9-1. The Tiers of Coverage

	Traditional Consumers	New Consumers
The Securely Enfranchised (Roughly 38% of total U.S. population) *Total U.S. population 1999 = 273,652,000*	▪ age 18 to 64, no college education, high-income workers (and spouses) with no PCs but high job security, with private managed care plans or fee-for-service insurance (paid by employers or self) ▪ age 65+, no college education, moderate to high savings/resources, no PCs, Medicare only or Medicare and private insurance ▪ children securely insured	▪ age 18 to 64, college-educated, high-income workers (and spouses) with high job security, with private managed care plans or fee-for-service insurance (paid by employers or by self) ▪ age 55 to 64, early retirees, college-educated, high savings/resources, private managed care plans or fee-for-service insurance (paid by generous former employers or by self) ▪ age 65+, college-educated, moderate to high savings/resources, with PCs, Medicare + private insurance ▪ children securely insured
The Insecurely Enfranchised (Roughly 34% of total U.S. population)	▪ age 18 to 64, no college education, low- to moderate-income workers (and spouses) with low job security, in managed care plans (paid by employers or military) ▪ age 55 to 64, early retirees, no college education, low to moderate incomes, in managed care plans (paid by former employers who are not reassuring about keeping retiree benefits, or have already tried to reduce them) ▪ children securely insured	▪ age 18 to 64, college-educated, middle-income workers (and spouses) with PCs and low job security, in managed care plans (paid by employers, by military, or by self) ▪ age 55 to 64, early retirees, college-educated, high incomes, in managed care plans (paid by former employers who are not reassuring about keeping retiree benefits, or have already tried to reduce them) ▪ age 18 to 54, no college education, high-income but low-job-security workers (and spouses), with PCs, in managed care plans (paid by employers) ▪ children securely insured
The Disenfranchised (Roughly 28% of total U.S. population)	▪ age 18 to 64, no college education, unemployed and/or very poor, uninsured or on Medicaid ▪ children uninsured ▪ children on Medicaid or other government assistance	▪ age 18 to 34, temporarily uninsured, some college, with PCs, no full-time job yet or between early low-income jobs

Source: IFTF.

FORECAST AND ASSUMPTIONS

THE BOTTOM TIER: THE DISENFRANCHISED

Forecast

Because they largely lack a college education and have less access to information, and because their energy is focused on issues of access to care, this tier is unlikely to drive a consumer revolution or to be greatly affected by one. Although this group has many reasons to protest, it lacks voice and clout. Their advocates may push for legislation, particularly to cover children, but as a bloc these consumers have relatively little power over government or employers—their voter participation rates are lower than average, some are unemployed, their incomes are low, and a sizable group are minorities who face discrimination in many arenas. If the problem of access is to be solved for this tier, the solution will likely be driven by advocacy groups and members of the other two tiers. A factor that might motivate some action from the top two tiers would be the spread of drug-resistant infectious diseases, exacerbated by lack of proper care, from the lower tier into the other two tiers.

Assumptions

■ Lack of access to information and resources is a significant barrier to empowerment.

■ Advocates for the bottom tier will be largely ineffective in changing legislation and the structure of care.

■ Struggling for access prevents people from putting energy into other aspects of empowerment.

■ The plight of the disenfranchised will not become so visibly horrible that it triggers the level of mass dissatisfaction with the health care system that would lead to comprehensive reform.

THE MIDDLE TIER: THE INSECURELY ENFRANCHISED

Forecast

The portion of new consumers in the middle tier and advocacy organizations representing them make up the first segment that will want the system to provide high-quality consumer-oriented information about performance. These middle-tier new consumers are a rapidly growing group—demographic factors are driving a steady transfer of people, about 2 percent a year, from the lower middle class into the new consumer group, and many of these are in the insecurely enfranchised middle tier.

Because benefits insecurity and worries about coverage and out-of-pocket costs are currently this group's major issues—and will be even more so in the predicted recession of 1999 to 2000—the first report cards have focused on the relative merits of health plans. Because many people in this tier work for small employers, however, many do not have a choice of plan. Thus employers initially will be the biggest market for this type of report card.

Report cards on plans are already stimulating demand for similar report cards on providers, to help both employers and their employees in this tier choose providers that offer the best value.

Because provider report cards are consistent with the cost-efficiency goals of

Chapter 9: Health Care Consumers   131

plans, plans will continue to pursue their development both for hospitals and medical groups and eventually perhaps for individual physicians. Providers will object to such report cards, but they will be given little choice in the matter.

The older people in this tier, particularly the early retirees, are half new and half traditional consumers. Although the traditional consumers may complain more than they did in the past as American culture shifts from passivity to active skepticism, they will not have enough access to information to narrow the patient–provider information gap much, and thus will not be in the best position to demand change in the organization of their care. They will, however, be very experienced with the system and motivated to improve their care. They also vote. Increasing their access to information would help them have a greater impact.

Health consumers who have not yet retired may be able to put some pressure on their employers to keep their pension health benefits intact, but their numbers are too small for their complaints to stimulate major change. Employers are more concerned with pleasing young, educated employees. Older consumers will be heard primarily through their high voting rates and through advocacy groups like the American Association of Retired Persons (AARP). Although advocacy groups may change public policy, they may have less effect on provider behavior.

When the voices of the elderly traditional consumer in the middle tier are combined with those of the aging new

consumers in the top two tiers, the elderly may be a major force for changes in the organization of care at both the provider and plan levels. As they get sicker, they will push for greater security of benefits and for greater flexibility, service, and coverage in managed care plans and from providers.

Assumptions
- Increased choice leads to increased need for information.
- Empowerment and access to information will be tightly linked.

THE TOP TIER: THE SECURELY ENFRANCHISED

Forecast

The aging upper-tier new consumers though relatively small in numbers now are growing rapidly as most of the baby boom generation turns 50 over the next decade. As these informed consumers begin to encounter the more chronic and severe illnesses that accompany advancing age, they will interact more frequently with providers and plans in demanding change. Indeed, they have already begun to drive a shift in the culture away from passive respect of providers and toward more active engagement in their care.

This segment will use all three major modes of empowerment: (1) choice of plans and providers; (2) ability to provide self-care and self-management of their chronic diseases; and (3) ability and desire to share medical decisions with their providers. By 2010, as the first of the baby boom cohort reaches 65, this group will have paved the way for a revolution in the organization of care—a revolution simultaneously being fomented in other sectors of the system, as noted in the other chapters of this report.

Because the new consumers in the top tier are information rich, and as health-related information sources like the Internet are growing rapidly, they are increasingly marshaling enough information to narrow the patient–provider information gap. They are not as preoccupied with benefits security as the new consumers in the middle tier are, so empowerment becomes their most pressing issue.

The youngest new consumers in this tier are not very sick and so many of them do not interact with providers with the frequency required to demand big changes. Some do, however, particularly women of childbearing age, who interact with providers both for OB/GYN care and on behalf of their children. Young men and women will focus their demands on better customer service from plans and greater access to more open networks of providers.

Although continued employer mediation of health plan choices will limit new consumers' direct impact on plans to some extent, today's employers do tend to listen to the needs of their young employees. New consumers will encounter health plan customer service issues simply in the process of signing up for plans and choosing or switching primary care providers. They will encounter provider interaction issues when undergoing routine exams. They will affect plans by complaining to their employers and pressuring employers to complain to the plans or switch to more

customer-friendly plans. Those new consumers who have a choice will simply switch. Because they are not sick enough to see very many providers very often, their effect on changing provider interactions and increasing shared decision making will be relatively small before 2010. Beyond 2010, these young new consumers will join the older group in driving a change toward patient-centered care.

In contrast to the young new consumers in this tier, the elderly are the sickest segment of the population, and they do interact frequently with providers. Most will purchase their care directly from providers and can take their Medicare money elsewhere if they don't like a particular provider. This gives them power in the health care market. Because the elderly are also a large voting bloc and have powerful lobbying organizations like the AARP, they are a potent force for both legislative and market change. Although we estimate that two-thirds of the elderly in the upper tier are traditional consumers whose impact on provider behavior will be greatly muted by their inability to bridge the information gap, even they will be influential in supporting legislation that protects their rights to privacy and dignity, especially in end-of-life medical decisions.

Both traditional and new elderly consumers in this tier will also be outlets for the voices of their adult children, many of whom are baby boomer new consumers. This baby boomer "sandwich generation"— especially the women— interacts with the health care system through both its children and its parents. These more assertive and informed baby boomers will attempt to intervene with providers as advocates for their parents, adding to the latter's impact. If large numbers of the traditional elderly consumers begin to switch providers or plans based on their children's advice, they will act as amplifiers of the voice of the new consumer. This amplified impact would be mostly in the direction of more patient-centered care and better service but to some degree, as some of the elderly have children in the middle tier, it might also push plans to address middle-tier issues by offering more coverage and better value.

Assumptions

- Health care legislation empowering patients will not be the primary force behind change in provider behavior and plans, although it may begin to have a larger effect as the baby boom generation ages and its voter participation increases.

- Most providers will not be motivated to bridge the patient–provider information gap, as that would reduce their power and status.

- Information technologies that would aid shared decision making (e.g., the EMR or smart databases) will be fairly slow to develop, limiting the development of the shared decision-making form of empowerment.

THREE LEVELS OF EMPOWERMENT WILL ARRIVE AT DIFFERENT TIMES

Of the three elements of consumer empowerment in health care, informed choice of providers and plans will develop first as middle- and upper-tier new consumers join forces with plans to create report cards. We estimate that roughly 10 percent to 15 percent of all people today have access to any information on plan quality. In some areas, such information is published in newspapers or on the Internet, but in most it is not yet available. We forecast that, by 2010, 50 percent of all consumers will have access to understandable comparative information on plan quality. Because networks will become increasingly more open, however, such information will become less and less useful over time. Provider report cards will be increasingly called for and are already being developed by some plans.

The other two elements of empowerment—self-care and shared decision making—depend more on the cooperation of providers, who right now are busy organizing themselves to resist the strictures being imposed on them by managed care. Of these two elements, self-care and self-management will be the next to emerge, in part because they will be assisted by pressures from plans to reduce costs. As the new consumers rapidly gain access to information, both online and through traditional media, they will narrow the patient–provider information gap and make effective self-care possible and desirable.

We forecast that, by 2010, 30 percent of health plan members will be able to identify the three most important threats to their health status, and a large proportion of these folks will be actively engaged in executing elements of their treatment plans. Right now, we estimate that only 5 to 10 percent of members engage in self-care or self-management. Medical technologies involving remote sensing of patients' vital signs will hasten this development.

Shared decision making will be the last element of consumer empowerment to take hold. Its tardy arrival is due partly to provider resistance to change and partly to the fact that many medical decisions are so complex that they require a sophisticated informational infrastructure to assist both patients and providers. This infrastructure will be slow to emerge. The issue of confidentiality of medical records may further slow the emergence of this infrastructure. The quality of medical information available on the Internet will also be a factor. We estimate that right now only 1 percent of consumers share decision making with their providers. We forecast that by 2010, 10 percent of all consumers will be aware of the primary treatment choices implicit in the health risks they face and will share with their providers decisions about treatment paths, the providers helping them to pick paths in line with their personal preferences and values. Consumers with chronic illnesses are likely to be at the forefront of this shift. This element of empowerment also has the most potential to transform the system in the longer term and improve health status.

On the down side, shared decision making, if widely implemented, may exacerbate the widening gap in access and health status between the information-rich new consumers and the information-poor traditional consumers. Information access is key to effective shared decision making. Ultimately, beyond 2010, this could push us toward a two-tier system in which the information "haves" have secure access to high-value, patient-centered care whereas the information "have-nots" struggle for access, choice, and value.

All of these facets add up to a forecast for incremental consumer-driven change by 2010—not a full-blown consumer revolution. Nonetheless, consumer forces will build rapidly in the growing top tier by 2010, and this will shift the passive consumer culture significantly in the direction of active skepticism. The combination of this shift, the push toward self-care by cost-conscious plans, patients' rights legislation supported by the elderly, and slow but steady improvements in the information infrastructure will prepare the way for a major consumer revolution when the baby boomers begin to hit age 65 in 2010 and beyond.

WILD CARDS

■ The "information poor" get "wired," gaining increased access to information through technologies like WebTV, and thus become part of the force for change.

■ Employers switch en masse to a defined contribution system, making defined benefits obsolete and putting health care purchasing back in the hands of patients, thus converting health care to a demand-driven system well before 2010.

- Biosensors and other new medical technologies reduce costs dramatically, rather than increasing them, and lead to do-it-yourself home care improving access in the process.

- Spillover of infectious diseases from a rapidly growing uninsured population into the middle and top tiers leads to national legislation to fix the safety net, shrinking the bottom tier.

- Congress and the president join forces to push through legislation to reduce benefits insecurity, shrinking the middle tier.

Congress and the president join forces to push Medicare entirely to HMOs or cut benefits drastically, shrinking the top tier—or igniting a revolution among the elderly.

ENDNOTE

[1] By "access to care" we do not mean convenience but rather ability to get even minimally adequate care when it is needed. This basic access is limited in this tier by inability to pay—either out of pocket, or for insurance —and by the poor quality and limited resources of the facilities available to those with limited ability to pay.

CHAPTER 10

Public Health Services

A Challenging Future

The goal of public health is to secure health and promote wellness, for both individuals and communities, by addressing the societal, environmental, and individual determinants of health. As defined by the WHO, health is "A state of complete well-being, physical, social, and mental, and not merely the absence of disease or infirmity."

Despite the merit of this intent, a lack of consensus on the public health mission, inadequate capacity in the field, disjointed decision making, hobbled leadership, and organizational fragmentation led the Institute of Medicine (IOM) in 1988 to liken public health to a "shattered vision." More than 10 years later, has that assessment borne out? What does the future of public health look like today, and what will it look like in the next decade?

This chapter highlights some of the public health issues in the United States, reviewing briefly the development of the public health system and identifying broad social, political, and technological forces that will shape its future.

THE HISTORY OF PUBLIC HEALTH IN THE UNITED STATES

The IOM describes the history of the public health system in the United States as "a history of bringing knowledge and values together in the public arena to shape an approach to health problems." By understanding the history of today's public health system, we may forecast how public health might look tomorrow.

Before the 18th century, disease was widely believed to be associated primarily with a person's moral standing. During the 18th century, there evolved a sentiment that disease could be prevented, and an organized health infrastructure began to develop. Galvanized by industrial urbanization, by a realization that both rich and poor were vulnerable to disease, and by the "great sanitary awakening" of the early 19th century, the shape of public health changed profoundly as society developed a dynamic strategy to prevent disease through public action and environmental hygiene. By the second half of the 19th century, public health was dramatically altered again as evolution of the germ theory grounded public health in science. (See Table 10-1.)

Table 10-1. Stages of Relations Between Public Health and Medicine

Period	Public Health	Medicine
Pre 20th century era of infectious disease: *Cooperation*	Focus on prevention: sanitary engineering, environmental hygiene, quarantine	Focus on treatment: direct patient care within comprehensive framework
Early 20th century era of bacteriology: *Professionalization*	Establishment of targeted disease control; Rockefeller Foundation report creates science-based schools of public health	Establishment of the biomedical model of disease, Flexner Report leading to standard science-based medical education
Post World War II era of biomedical paradigm: *Functional separation*	Focus on behavioral risk factors, development of publicly funded medical safety net (Medicaid/Medicare)	Pursuit of biological mechanisms of heart disease, cancer, and stroke, success with pharmacology, diagnostics, therapeutic procedures

Source: IFTF; Lasker, R., and the Committee on Medicine and Public Health of the New York Academy of Medicine. *Medicine and Public Health: The Power of Collaboration.* New York: NYAM, 1997.

Before the germ theory was propagated, public health's efforts at disease control aimed to improve living conditions through environmental hygiene, whereas medical efforts focused on individual treatment by private physicians. There was a great deal of interdependence between the two. With acceptance of the germ theory, the new domains of public health and private medicine could no longer be readily distinguished, as population health interventions—such as screening, immunization, and the treatment of communicable disease—were provided to individuals, usually in a physician's office. Problems deepened with the creation of the health care safety net that assigned to the public sector medical responsibility for patients unable to obtain care in the private sector. Whereas the public sector had traditionally addressed the health of the population, it was now to provide a mixture of population and personal health services.

With this change, the responsibility for public health progressively was placed in the hands of professional health experts, and programs were instituted that focused on specific disease transmission routes, established immunization programs and water sanitation as cornerstones of disease prevention, and expanded governmental participation in public health efforts.

The blurring of the distinction between population-based disease prevention and individual-based medical treatment extended into the 20th century. Roosevelt's New Deal in the 1930s and Johnson's Great Society programs in the 1960s served as bookends for the expansion of the federal role in health planning, promotion, education, and financing. With the Social Security Act and the Medicare and Medicaid programs, public health moved away from population-based approaches and became more involved in individual interventions. As health care costs increased and the resulting economic burden became unbearable, the social vision again changed as the focus turned to cost con-

Figure 10-1. Changes in Cause of Death , 1900–1999

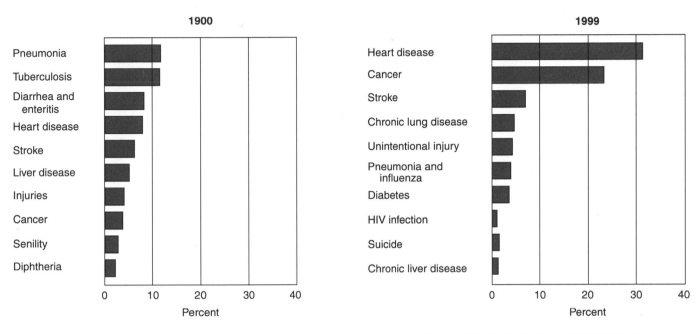

Source: Centers for Disease Control and Prevention. Control of infectious diseases, 1900–1999. *Morbidity and Mortality Weekly Report* 1999; 48:621–629.

tainment. The last decades of the 20th century ushered in the managed care system of health care delivery and further diminished support for a population-based public health infrastructure.

Table 10-2. Ten Public Health Achievements, 1900–1999

Vaccination
Motor vehicle safety
Safer workplaces
Control of infectious diseases
Decline in deaths from coronary heart disease and stroke
Safer and healthier foods
Healthier mothers and babies
Family planning
Fluoridation of drinking water
Recognition of tobacco use as a health hazard

Source: Centers for Disease Control and Prevention. Ten great public health achievements—United States, 1900–1999. *Morbidity and Mortality Weekly Report* 1999; 48:241–243.

PUBLIC HEALTH ACHIEVEMENTS IN THE 20TH CENTURY

Over the course of the century, infectious diseases diminished as a major cause of morbidity and mortality while chronic disease and behavioral health risks grew. The 20th century brought Americans improved health and longevity, their life expectancy lengthening by 30 years since 1900.[1] According to the Centers for Disease Control and Prevention (CDC), 25 of those years can be attributed to advances in public health, which accomplished ten significant achievements during the 20th century (see Table 10-2).

There is much cause for celebration over the accomplishments of the 20th century, and yet much still needs to be done. (See Figure 10-1.)

PUBLIC HEALTH STRUCTURE AND FUNCTION TODAY

The mission of public health, as viewed by the IOM, is the use of knowledge to fulfill the public's interest in reducing human suffering and enhancing quality of life. The substance of this mission lies in organized community efforts that are aimed at the prevention of disease and the promotion of health. These efforts are guided by public health principles, which include a scientific basis for action, an orientation toward prevention of illness and promotion of wellness, a population-wide perspective, community-based participation and problem solving, and a respect for diversity. Ideally, these efforts and principles are applied within an organizational framework that encompasses governmental, private, voluntary, and individual activities.

The U.S. government is at the core of the public health system, acting as the primary source of leadership and accountability. The IOM delineates three functional pillars of public health that the government should guarantee: assessment, policy development, and assurance (see Figure 10-2).

Involvement of the federal government in public health efforts fluctuated during the 20th century. At the close of the century, federal intervention had been retracted, although the role of the federal government continued to be important because of its capacity to address interstate and international health issues, to develop overarching national health policy, and to coordinate national health data and research. State governments now have the greatest responsibility for the well-being of the state's residents, not only because of the reductions in federal intervention but also because of their constitutionally designated police powers. It is local government that is on the front line of public health action today, however. Local governments are critical to the public health system, providing an operational mechanism for public health action and serving as a liaison among professional experts, different governmental divisions, and the community.

Myriad other institutions contribute to public health practice, including private foundations, schools of public health, community-based organizations, private health care organizations, and community activist organizations. In this diversity of public health players lie both opportunity and challenge. Opportunity because public health problems tend to be complex and require integrated, multidisciplinary responses. Challenge because these various players can be uncoordinated and even competitive in their efforts.

KEY FACTORS AFFECTING PUBLIC HEALTH IN AMERICA TODAY

POLITICS: THE AMERICAN DREAM UNDER RECONSTRUCTION

The mid-20th century was a time of expansion of prosperity and the American dream, but the recessions of the 1970s and 1980s and government downsizing in the 1990s narrowed the government's social vision. Welfare and affirmative action receded. Government privatized the safety net, borrowed from Social

Figure 10-2. The Three Pillars of Public Health

Assessment

The diagnosis of community health status and needs through epidemiology, surveillance, research, and evaluation of information about disease, behavioral, biological, environmental, and socioeconomic factors.

Policy Development

Planning and priority setting, based on scientific knowledge and under the leadership of the governmental agency, for the development of comprehensive public health policies and decision making.

Assurance

The securing of universal access to a set of essential personal and community-wide health services through delegation, regulation, or direct public provision of services.

Evaluation

Source: Institute of Medicine, Division of Health Care Services, 1988.

Security, and embraced free trade. Government spending on infrastructure, education, and research has diminished from 24 percent of the federal budget to 14 percent over the past 25 years.[2]

Yet, at the end of the 20th century, new health challenges emerged, such as AIDS infection and environmental contamination, that required strong centralized leadership and reintegration of population-based approaches to public health.

Two currents now flow through the mainstream, and one of them is likely to dominate in shaping the next social vision. One current is simultaneously populist, equitable, libertarian, pro-

environment, fiscally conservative, and intrinsically supportive of effective public spending for social good. The other is fiscally conservative, characterized by market populism, and oriented toward increased privatization that would intrinsically limit government's involvement in health reforms.

The first political vision is fundamentally new, and the policies it would deliver are less certain. The second vision would definitely restrict government establishment of such policies as universal health coverage, a patient's bill of rights, and overall increases in social, health, and public health spending.

SOCIOECONOMIC AND POLITICAL FACTORS

Socioeconomic status is the number one predictor of poor health. The poor are more than three times as likely as the wealthy to die prematurely or have a disability from illness,[3] despite nearly two-thirds of the money for public health being directed to medical safety-net services.[2] Socioeconomic status is a powerful factor among the determinants of intentional injury by homicide and suicide. The issue is clearly socioeconomic status and not ethnicity because when rates of household crowding are used as an index of socioeconomic status, African Americans are no more likely to commit domestic homicide than are whites in comparable socioeconomic circumstances.[4] The ill effects of poverty are particularly ominous in the light of an increasing economic gap between the rich and poor, which is independently associated with a worse health status for the bottom economic tiers of society.

Chapter 10: Public Health Services

Economic disparity in the United States has increased over the past two decades. From 1977 to 1999, the after-tax income for the richest 1 percent of the population increased 115 percent, whereas the after-tax income for the poorest 20 percent declined by 9 percent[5] (see Figure 10-3). Moreover, greater wealth is concentrated in a smaller segment of society today than has been the case at any time since the Great Depression. This disparity will have as large an effect on the future of public health as any other factors considered in this analysis.

GLOBAL FORCES DRIVING AND LIMITING PROGRESS

Global issues ultimately create the context for public health today and into the future. They are highly integrated economic, social, political, and technological forces that both drive and inhibit progress.

The world's economies are interconnected more than ever before, and the advent of free-trade agreements and expanded world travel are rapidly changing the context of public health in the United States. The main mechanism through which globalism is shaping public health is through the breakdown of natural and regulatory barriers to disease. Increased trade and travel are permitting diseases to spread to new populations that have no natural resistance and organisms to enter new environments with no natural controls.

These forces of globalism are inevitably associated with health risks, including new infectious diseases, contaminated food, spread of emerging and drug-resistant disease, bioterrorism, and toxic substances, both legal and illegal. According to CDC, since 1995, nearly 50 percent of all cases of measles reported in the United States have been introduced from other countries,[6] as have been the influenza strains that affect the U.S. population every year. In 1997, 39 percent of all patients with tuberculosis reported in the United States, and 67 percent in California, were foreign born.[7] An increasing proportion of the foods Americans eat, including 40 percent of fruits and 60 percent of seafood, is produced abroad, where standards of pesticide use and sanitation can differ from the United States.[8]

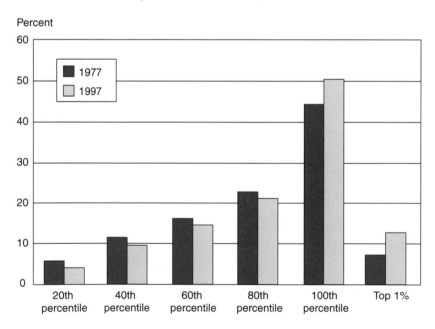

Figure 10-3. Changes in the Share of National After-Tax Income Held by Various Economic Groups in the United States, 1977 and 1997

Source: IFTF; Shapiro, I., and Greenstein, R. *The Widening Income Gap*. Washington, DC: Center on Budget and Policy Priorities, 1999.

International free trade is also challenging national and state health and safety regulations. The primary issue is how to maintain and advance U.S. health and environmental standards without violating trade accords and while remaining competitive. Reconciling this issue from a public health perspective will be like walking a tightrope, with liability and environmental and health risks all in the balance. For example, the Vancouver-based Methanex Corporation may sue the State of California if the legislature enacts a planned ban against the gasoline additive methyltertiary butyl ether (MTBE), claiming violation of NAFTA.[9] MTBE has extensively contaminated groundwater in California, although it was once considered a panacea for refineries attempting to meet Clean Air Act requirements.

The next 10 years will see increasing international cooperation in vaccine preparation, disease control, and environmental and food safety. The reality and the perception of public health concerns and solutions in the United States 10 years from now will be much more embedded in a global health and economic context. Policymakers and public health professionals will increasingly be called upon to protect the public and the environment in a way that both withstands the pressures and advances with the opportunities of global trade.

ENVIRONMENTAL FACTORS

A fragmentation of the infrastructure and information systems that supported environmental health until the last quarter of the 20th century has weakened the ability of public health agencies to protect the communities they serve. While there are ample data available, there is little usable information—a factor that has proved to be a serious barrier to public health agencies' ability to address emerging health problems, to educate decision makers and the public about specific environmental hazards, and to evaluate the effectiveness of interventions.[10]

The next 10 years will see public health professionals in the environmental health field creating multisectoral relationships like never before. Their success in creating links to government environmental agencies, environmental activist groups, human rights groups, labor unions, and technology agencies will be one of the primary determinants of the status of environmental health in the United States over the coming decade.

Three major areas will be of greatest importance: air quality, water quality, and food safety.

Air Quality

The good news is that Los Angeles no longer has the worst air quality in the nation. While California has broken new ground with air quality improvements, particularly in regard to motor vehicle emissions, other states have continued to pollute their air. The most important concerns in this area are the improvement of vehicular, diesel, industrial (especially power), and household product emissions.

The bad news is that failure to improve air quality has profound repercussions on health, including its relation to cancer, developmental problems, and asthma.

Asthma is one of the most common chronic diseases in the United States and

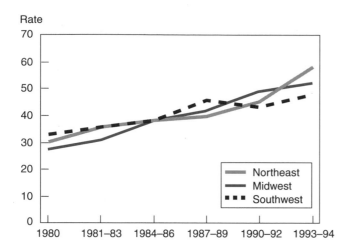

Figure 10-4. Trends in Asthma Prevalence by Region and Year, 1980–1994

Source: Mannino, D. M., et al. Surveillance for asthma—United States, 1960–1995. *Morbidity and Mortality Weekly Report* 1998; 47 (SS-1):1–28.

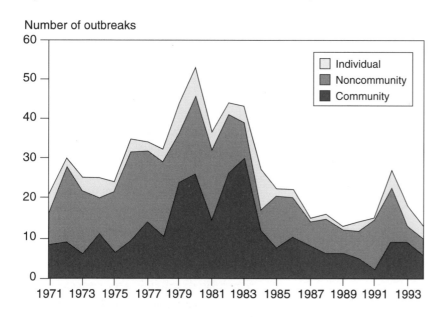

Figure 10-5. Trends in Waterborne Disease Outbreaks, 1971–1994

Source: Centers for Disease Control and Prevention. Surveillance for waterborne disease outbreaks—United States, 1993–1994. *Morbidity and Mortality Weekly Report* 1996; 45 (SS-1):1–33.

is the ninth leading cause of hospitalization nationally. Despite medical advancements in its diagnosis and treatment, the prevalence rates linked to asthma are increasing nationally, and overall rates of death with asthma as the underlying cause—which decreased from 1962 through 1977—have gradually increased again in all race, sex, and age strata. From 1980 to 1994, the prevalence of self-reported asthma in the United States increased 75 percent (see Figure 10-4). An estimated 17 million people in the United States had asthma in 1998, representing almost a 20 percent increase from the already high levels of 1994, and signifying prevalence rates of 5.8 to 7.2 percent. The most substantial increases occurred among children from infancy to 14 years of age.[11,12] Allergic asthma costs an estimated $6.2 billion a year, according to the National Institute of Environmental Health Science.

Water Quality

Most attention to water quality has focused on drinking water, as public water systems are regulated under the federal Safe Drinking Water Act of 1974, as amended in 1986. Probably as a result of this regulation, the number of waterborne disease outbreaks reported annually has been similar for each year from 1987 through 1994, except for an increase in 1992[13] (see Figures 10-5 and 10-6). Some recent outbreaks have disclosed the vulnerability of large metropolitan areas. However, the capacity to treat drinking water adequately in some metropolitan areas is being stretched to its limit, and the problem cannot necessarily be remedied by further regulation. As a consequence, municipalities increas-

Figure 10-6. Patterns in Waterborne Disease Outbreaks, 1993–1994

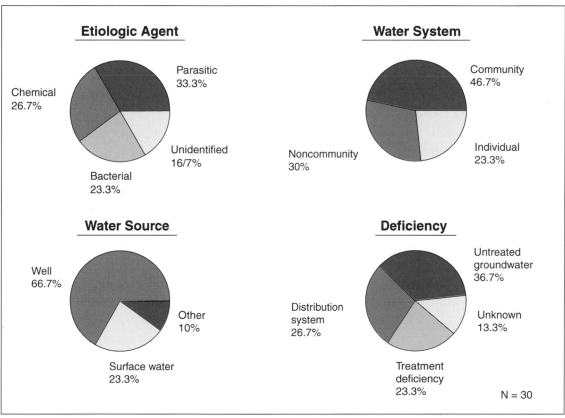

Source: Centers for Disease Control and Prevention. Surveillance for waterborne disease outbreaks—
United States, 1993–1994. *Morbidity and Mortality Weekly Report* 1996; 45 (SS-1):1–33.

ingly will explore new technologies in water sanitation.

Two other sources of water contamination are also emerging areas for concern. According to the Environmental Protection Agency, farm animal waste produced at concentrated animal feeding operations has polluted 35,000 miles of rivers in 22 states and has contaminated groundwater in 17 states. Animal-factory pollution contributes to a range of physical and mental ailments in people, including headaches, nausea, depression,

and even death. The practice of feeding animals large quantities of antibiotics also contributes to drug-resistant bacterial infections. Although the number of hog farms in the United States has dropped from 600,000 to 157,000 over the past 15 years, the total hog inventory for the United States has remained constant because of the increased animal concentration in large-scale farms. Securing water safety in the future will require structural, regulatory, or redesign interventions in this domain.

The second area of concern is increasing evidence of microcontaminants and pharmaceuticals in water supplies. Hormone-disrupting contaminants such as DDT-like compounds and waterborne perchlorate as well as other pesticides are of particular importance. An emerging issue is that greater than expected quantities of active pharmaceuticals are turning up in water, in large part excreted by humans who have not entirely metabolized the medicines that they take. In some cases, 50 to 90 percent of an administered drug may be excreted.[14] Drugs, however, are not traditionally considered pollutants and are regulated primarily by public health agencies that have little expertise in protecting natural ecosystems and water supplies. The full impact of pharmaceuticals in the water supply is only beginning to emerge and may prompt new standards for drug approval and cross-sector collaboration in their control.

Food Safety

Two main areas of concern in food safety are outbreaks related to foodborne pathogens and pesticide use.

Each year, millions of people have a foodborne illness, but because only a fraction of them seek medical care and even fewer submit laboratory specimens, estimates of the magnitude of foodborne illness in the United States are imprecise. Since 1996, however, the Foodborne Diseases Active Surveillance Network (FoodNet) has collected data to monitor nine foodborne diseases at selected sites in the United States. As compared to the 1996 data, 1998 FoodNet data indicate a decline in several of the major bacterial and parasitic causes of foodborne illness[15] (see Figure 10-7). These declines might in part reflect annual fluctuations, temporal variations in diagnostic practices, or implementation of disease prevention regulations. However, with the forces of increased international food trade and increased fast-food consumption, constant vigilance over this system is required to secure ongoing declines.

Pesticide use has implications for both food consumption and environmental or occupational exposure. Certain pesticides are known carcinogens, and others are under suspicion. Of particular concern is that these chemicals can be excreted in breast milk and that children consume the greatest concentration of pesticides. Mounting evidence shows that when children are exposed to ambient pesticides through proximity in or outside their home, their normal physical and intellectual development are profoundly affected. In adults, occupational exposure can be associated with bradycardia, diaphoresis, nausea, headache, eye irritation, or muscle weakness, as well as with a potential for more severe effects, including cancer, over the long term. Again, international differences in agricultural practices as well as trade agreements are major considerations in addressing these problems.

The Future of Air, Water, and Food Safety

In all cases of air, water, and food safety, it is children and developing fetuses who have the most adverse health consequences of environmental threats. Growing evidence to this effect has created an increasing momentum to change the way environmental health and safety standards are set. Within 10 years, the gold standard for setting levels for contami-

Figure 10-7. Rates of Foodborne Disease Incidence, 1996–1998

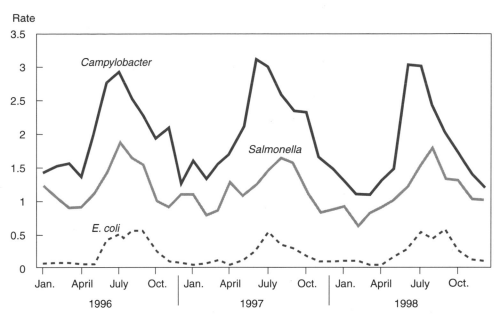

Source: Centers for Disease Control and Prevention. Incidence of foodborne illnesses. *Morbidity and Mortality Weekly Report* 1999; 48:189–194.

nants will be based on child health factors, with important implications for trade and industry. International accords will have as great a role in the setting of environmental standards as will the work of national and state governments. The global context will require environmental health professionals to think in new ways and build alliances across environmental, labor, and technology sectors.

TECHNOLOGY

Technological advancements are so frequent and often dramatic now that change itself seems to be commonplace. Technology holds the greatest implications for public health in the areas of information, diagnostics, and genetic technologies. New information technolo-

gies are expanding public health's capacity to conduct epidemiology, disease surveillance, collaborative research, data-based policymaking, and advocacy. At the same time, tremendous struggles regarding privacy and data ownership, validity, and coordination have yet to be resolved.

Diagnostic technologies will continue to advance public health screening. New technologies include more sensitive mammograms, noninvasive screening with enzyme-linked immunoabsorbant assays and polymerase chain reaction tests, and computer-aided detection of abnormalities on pap smears and mammograms. These advances permit more and better screening, and also make it easier to screen in nontraditional settings, such as jails and community outreach sites, allowing access to otherwise hard-to-reach populations.

With progress in our understanding of genetic predispositions to disease, the implications for public health screening and epidemiology are impressive. However, biotechnology also ushers in a new array of ethical struggles, as debate ignites issues of stem-cell research, genetic screening, and international trials. Technology also helps drive the increase in resources expended on health care, further diminishing the funds available for public health services.

PUBLIC HEALTH FRAMEWORKS AND STRATEGIES: PROBLEMS OF PERCEPTION

PUBLIC HEALTH AS THE "ALSO RAN"

Ask most people on the street what public health means and they'll tell you, "welfare." Ask them what epidemiology means and they'll either blush or tell you it's the study of skin infections. Public health has an identity problem.

People often think of public health as publicly funded medical care for the poor. But while medicine and public health are inextricably entwined, they are also quite distinct. A physician's virtual black bag contains diagnostic tools, pharmaceuticals, treatments, and protocols. A public health professional's toolkit carries epidemiology and biostatistics, health education, program and policy development and evaluation,

screening, and advocacy. Americans can see what doctors do any night of the week on television, but they have almost no exposure to what public health professionals do. This lack of understanding of public health can forestall reinvigoration of the public health system.

Furthermore, while people value the protections offered by public health, they do not know what it takes to achieve those protections. People value the *products* of public health, such as clean water, a clean environment, and control of communicable disease, but they do not as greatly value the *methods* of public health, such as disease surveillance and screening. The better public health's prevention strategies work, the more invisible they are to the public's eye. Ultimately, if the public does not value and support the means to the end, things will fall apart.

Two tendencies, one reactive and one active, indicate that improvements in public awareness are possible. Resurgence in public support for public health reforms does occur, but largely as reaction to a perceived crisis. It took 45,000 stray dogs and an epidemic of dog bites for Los Angeles County recently to reverse an 8-year trend of funding cuts to its animal control program. It has taken numerous mass shootings to galvanize the public and convince some politicians to take steps toward gun control. It may require a worsening of problems, such as drug-resistant tuberculosis or breaches in water-supply sanitation by microcontaminants, before the public becomes convinced that public health is not just for people on the outskirts of society, but rather is necessary for the well-being of the entire population. Public health professionals need to realize that embedded in these dilemmas are opportunities for heightening public awareness and support.

On a more positive note, another emerging trend—the rise of the "new consumer"—could put public health on the radar screen before disaster strikes. The new consumers not only are educated, they also have economic clout and are very well-informed about their health. With mounting exposure to public health information, the new consumers, if guided and organized, will serve as the opinion leaders necessary for enhancing the reputation and resources of public health. Moreover, these information-empowered consumers will become the majority of the adult population around 2005, and will bring with them a greater value for prevention (see Chapter 9).

ORGANIZATIONAL AND INSTITUTIONAL FORCES

Issues of public health leadership and professionalism, the organizational structure of public health, and public-private competition and accountability all influence the day-to-day functioning of the public health system. They also influence the potential for policy formation that could alter the course of public health in the future.

Public Health Professionalism: A Crisis of Leadership

Organizational factors that limit public health agencies' capacity to provide the leadership necessary to guarantee the three pillars of public health include uncompetitive wages, restrictive bureau-

cracies, and insufficient leadership training. Governmental public health officials' average wages are half those in medical and health services management and are less than one-third those of physicians.[16] Increasingly, public health practice relies on highly skilled professional staff, including epidemiologists, policy analysts, project directors, and information systems experts. Systemwide low salaries impair public health agencies' ability to compete for talented personnel.

Compounding the problem is the administrative structure of public health agencies, which is not always well suited to a professional staff. Restrictive job classifications, restrictions on recruitment and hiring, out-of-date time management requirements, and outmoded or counterproductive administration of professional positions can make public health an uncompetitive field. Unlike the private sector, the public sector is also restricted in its ability to reward highly productive employees or lay off underachieving employees.

Show Me the Money

Inadequate funding is one of the greatest barriers to the completion of public health's mission and responsibilities. At all levels of government, but particularly the local level, officials are hamstrung by limited funding and are often forced to follow the money rather than address public health problems. Although states have been given considerable flexibility in their use of block grants, this restrictive funding mechanism has often compromised the ability of local agencies to meet the particular needs of their communities, especially as the grants are not discretionary.

Chapter 10: Public Health Services

Organizational Challenges to Public Health

The states have considerable latitude in fulfilling their public health mission. Partly because of that autonomy, the organizational structures of different states' public health agencies and their ties to related agencies vary widely. Although greater uniformity is neither likely nor necessarily desirable, organizational variability can impede integration and coordination of health and social services.

A particular difficulty lies in creating functional organizational ties between public health and other agencies with overlapping missions, such as social services, environmental protection, environmental health, personal health care, and mental health agencies. When a new health problem emerges, health systems sometimes create organizational barriers, establishing a separate program for it rather than integrating that program into the existing infrastructure, as was the case with AIDS. The consequences of these barriers can include lack of coordination of program activities and policy priorities, inadequate and out-of-date data surveillance and information sharing, and competition for limited resources. The same problems exist between the government and private sectors, especially with the institution of managed care.

RECONCILING PUBLIC HEALTH AND PRIVATE MEDICINE

Perhaps the most significant example of an organizational threat to public health efficacy involves the interplay of the public and private sectors in the provision of personal health services. With the spectacular biomedical discoveries and their applications in the late 20th century has come expansion of the private medical sector, with concomitant further reductions in financial and public support of population-based public health programs and training. To this day, although the interests of public health and medicine overlap, an adequate mechanism for coordinating activities between the two sectors is lacking.

The problems resulting from this arrangement continue to weaken the public health system and are fourfold.

First, the disproportionate allocation of public health resources to publicly funded medicine drains capacity and attention from community-wide public service, assessment, and policy development functions. At the state level, two-thirds of spending is for personal health services whereas spending for population-based health services is only 1.0 percent of total health care expenditures. Of this, the largest amount (26 percent) is for enforcing laws and regulations that protect the health and ensure the safety of the public, whereas training (4 percent) and research (2 percent) received the smallest investments.[17]

Second, in both the public and private sectors, there is limited cooperation and coordination across public and personal health services for the provision of essential disease control functions. These services include screening, disease reporting, partner notification and treatment, treatment standardization, and diagnostic and treatment technology updates.

Third, opening of Medicaid and Medicare reimbursements to the private sector has reduced the resources available to state and local public health agencies. Initially, the public sector was able to support some of its infrastructure and provide care to the indigent through relatively high Medicaid reimbursements. Paradoxically, when private providers became eligible for those reimbursements, they successfully siphoned off the majority of reimbursement income and the healthiest patients, leaving the public sector with the burden of the indigent population but without the Medicaid/Medicare income. Moreover, private-sector involvement did not fundamentally increase health care coverage for the poor. As a result, the cash-strapped public health agencies are left providing medical care for the poor and provide little public health care for the overall population.

Fourth, as the government's public health agency became increasingly involved with the provision of medical care, the general public came to confuse public health with publicly funded medical services—with welfare. The consequence of the public's misunderstanding of the core functions of public health has diminished public support or sense of collective responsibility for public health actions. Some public health professionals even suggest that the public health field should change its name to population health to clarify things!

PRIVATIZATION: THE PROMISE OF PARTNERSHIPS

Market forces that affect the delivery of health care are significantly changing the financial base and functional role of pub-

lic health agencies. With the emergence of managed care, the trend toward downsizing governmental agencies, and the overall reductions in public health funding, public health agencies have increasingly turned toward developing leaner, more efficient delivery systems. In particular, they have begun exploring "privatization" as a potential community-based approach for assuring delivery of necessary public health services. Table 10-3 reviews findings from a recent Public Health Foundation review of the privatization experience.[18]

However, when Medicaid and Medicare patients leave the public sector to enter private-sector care, public health loses control over some of the services it has traditionally assured its patients. For example, Medicaid recipients, as a medically vulnerable population, often require "wraparound" care that provides services, such as transportation or translation services, that help them gain access to or communicate with their medical provider. Currently, when patients leave the public sector to enter private managed care programs, essential wraparound services are not uniformly provided. The capacity of government agencies to assess the public's health status, expenditures, and disease control measures is significantly altered when patients enter the capitated world of private managed care.

The increasing delivery of health services in managed care environments is of particular concern for the poor, but is also of relevance to the general population. Between 1985 and 1998, the proportion of HMO members enrolled in investor-owned plans increased sharply from 26 percent to 62 percent. Between 1980

Table 10-3. Factors in the Process of Privatizing Publicly Funded Public and Personal Health Services

Measure	Finding
Reasons for privatization	Implementation of state Medicaid waivers
	Effort to achieve cost savings and address fiscal concerns
	Downsizing and reorganizing government
	Effort to improve quality and efficiency
Barriers	Personnel issues
	Philosophical differences
	Difficulty in finding able or willing partners in the private sector
Facilitators	Involved community
	Maintenance of the government's role in core functions of assessment, policy development, and assurance
	Public health agencies' savvy in corporate skills and collaboration
	History of partnering
	Strong local health department leadership
Outcomes	Public health agencies maintain service delivery components related to assurance and ultimate accountability
	Little impact on quality of services, except in the case of access, where access increases for clinical service and decreases for psychological services and health education
	Health departments evaluate and redirect revenues and expenditures regardless of privatization, although privatization allows them to focus on essential public health
	Privatization strengthens community relations, but occasionally can weaken them

Source: IFTF; *Privatization and Public Health: A Study of Initiatives and Early Lessons Learned.* Washington, DC: Public Health Foundation, September 1997. Research and writing supported by The Annie E. Casey Foundation, Baltimore, Maryland.

and 1998, the market share of group-model and staff-model plans decreased from 81 percent to 12 percent. A recent study analyzing differences between for-profit and not-for-profit health plans found that investor-owned HMOs deliver a lower quality of care than do the not-for-profit plans. Compared with not-for-profit HMOs, investor-owned plans had lower rates for all 14 health plan employer data and information set (HEDIS) quality-of-care indicators. In particular, the investor-owned plans score lower in treatment of critical med-ical conditions and preventive health measures. Investor-owned plans had lower rates of immunization (63.9 versus 72.3 percent), mammography (69.4 versus 75.1 percent), Papanicolaou tests (69.2 versus 77.1 percent), and psychiatric hospitalization (70.5 versus 77.1 percent). Staff-model and group-model HMOs had higher scores on virtually all quality-of-care indicators.[19]

Public health involvement in the reconciliation of these concerns has focused on increasing efforts to negotiate shared

Chapter 10: Public Health Services

responsibilities either through government mandate or partnerships. Public-private partnerships are, to this date, the most prominent and perhaps most promising vehicle for guaranteeing governmental assurance and assessment responsibilities and for transforming managed care settings into productive protagonists for public health. Through public-private partnerships, the local public health agency can engage the private sector and community representatives in building healthy communities.

Experimentation with several models is currently under way, including models serving the underinsured and the uninsured together with patients enrolled in Medicare and private programs. For example, Medicaid primary care case management interlaces managed care and FFS health services as an alternative to the traditional HMO model. Introduced in Texas in 1996, it has already enrolled two-thirds of the state's eligible enrollees and may become the mainstream in other states as well. Such an arrangement fulfills the assurance function of the public health agency and streamlines the agency's assessment function as an added benefit to the community.

OTHER INSTITUTIONS: THE BREADTH OF PUBLIC HEALTH

Universities

University graduate schools of public health are, in a sense, the caretakers of the public health heritage. These schools train future public health professionals, provide technical support to government agencies, conduct basic research to further scientific understanding of health determinants, and provide leadership in

public health ethics and health and human rights issues. In so doing, they are a force that can standardize and shape the skills, principles, capacity, and knowledge of public health professionals at all levels.

Public health schools have an important role in shaping the future of public health. While there is a need for academics and researchers in public health, it is critical also to prepare future public health officials with skills in leadership, management, and negotiation. As a substantial proportion of current public health officials lack formal public health training and are resistant to efforts to further professionalize the field, more schools might follow the lead of schools that are developing distance education programs and creating nondegree certification programs.

Community-Based Organizations and Foundations

These organizations have the capacity to set political and program agendas through grassroots actions and financing of new initiatives. Community-based organizations are key members of any public-private partnership, as they are often among the strongest voices of constituency groups and can also provide services directly. Lack of funding consistently plagues community-based organizations, and innovative funding and public-private financing partnerships will have to be developed in the future. The potential for conflicts of interest resulting from new financing schemes will have to be evaluated. While community-based organizations seek funding, the foundations provide funding, and in so doing they play a leadership role in setting public health agendas and coordinating public health action.

THE FUTURE: SCENARIOS AND FORECASTS

OUTLOOK FOR PUBLIC-PRIVATE PARTNERSHIPS IN PERSONAL HEALTH CARE

There are three possible scenarios and three sets of key players whose leadership, management skills, and negotiation capabilities would predict the likelihood of particular scenario's occurrence. The three players determining the outlook for public-private relationships in personal health care include:

- public health agency directors
- private health care providers and organizations
- community-based organizations and leaders

Together, these players will lead their constituents through one of the following three scenarios.

Scenario One: Public-Private Community Partnerships

In this scenario, the medical services now provided by most government agencies are shifted to the private sector through a variety of public-private partnerships. The public health principles—especially those of prevention, shared standards and objectives, and community-based participation—potentiate this partnership. Public health agencies maintain a watchdog role to assure that vulnerable populations are served, but their focus returns primar-

ily to assessment, policy development, and population-level interventions, such as health systems monitoring or monitoring of food and water sanitation systems.

Scenario Two: Dynamic Competition Rules

Local public health agencies continue to provide medical services, successfully competing with the private sector for both Medicaid and private pay patients. Competition is both dynamic and effective and is confined to the provision of medical services. In this area, the advances and achievements in each sector drive improvements in the other's services. For example, the public sector's success in providing wraparound services pushes the private sector to improve its own services in this area. Most of the larger public health functions are provided by the public sector, although the private sector does join in to some extent for the sake of positive public relations.

Scenario Three: Public Health in Tatters

Unable to compete directly with the private sector or to develop successful partnerships, local public health agencies retreat from the provision of medical services, leaving only a skeleton framework of services remaining in order to fulfill their minimum mandates. The private sector serves all of the insured population, leaving the government health care systems strapped for cash. Without the revenues generated from Medicaid reimbursements and with no additional funding, the public health functions of assessment, policy development, and assurance are in tatters. The "invisible" work of public health, such as water and

156   Chapter 10: Public Health Services

food safety, becomes very visible as public health systems begin to fail and outbreaks and epidemics spread across the country. In some areas, community leaders begin to assist public health organizations through the private nonprofit sector.

FORECAST OF THE FUTURE: ORGANIZATIONAL ISSUES

The future of public health promises great struggle as public health leaders work to reinvigorate the infrastructure, approaches, and public attitudes that support a collective responsibility for society's well-being. It is not a question of whether there will be a future for public health—as long as people live together in society, public health will exist. Rather, the future asks the questions of how much, for how many, and how well?

Such questions are not easily answered at present. Money is short, organizing social vision is weak, and there predominates a sense that public health is relevant only to the poor. Our forecasts are based in this context. Nevertheless, there always exists the opportunity to challenge the future. We hope that, within these forecasts, public health professionals will see opportunities to shape a new era of public health that reaches its full potential to secure health for all.

During most of the next decade, public health will continue to be underfunded and marginalized, and for the most part efforts to address the underlying problems will be incremental. Breaches in public health prevention systems will

also become increasingly evident in the areas of food and water safety, air pollution, outbreaks of drug-resistant infections, and resurgence of sexually transmitted disease. As a result of these pressures, however, we think that government will begin to augment funding and pay attention to these systems.

Beyond the pressures of dysfunction, there are several key determinants of public health's future. These include the status of community health needs and community awareness, the relationship of the public health agency to the larger community, and the capacity of both the public and private sector to provide adequate personal health services to the community. Key public health actions will utilize policy, epidemiology, technology, public-private community coalitions, and information-empowered consumers. These are areas where focused energy will yield the greatest return.

IN PARTICULAR . . .

- *Community coalitions.* Coalitions establishing formal cooperative ties between community groups, private business, private health care agencies, community activists, and the government's health agency will become increasingly common during the next decade. Ideally led by a public health official, these coalitions will be a powerful vehicle for building healthy communities. Their approach will be to develop collaborative initiatives that mutually benefit business and community. Their function for public health will be to monitor and assure access to basic personal and public health services, to verify their quality, and to provide some support to cash-strapped community-based organizations. It is possible that up to 45 percent of public health departments will be engaged in some type of public-private partnership by the year 2010.

- Managed care. While apparently destined to be the dominant Medicaid personal health care model for this decade, up to 25 percent of public health agencies still will compete with the private marketplace to provide direct services to patients. Nevertheless, managed care will look different at the end of the decade than it does today. Competition and fiscal viability are continuing to drive innovation and experimentation. Patients' rights are going to be increasingly protected, which will also force managed care to either respond or fold. Think integration: of public and private partnerships, of insured and uninsured populations, and of managed care and FFS.

- Public health policy. At the national level, public health policy will approach assurance functions primarily in a piecemeal fashion but will include development of a patient's bill of rights and experimentation with safety-net incentive strategies. At the state level, the states will be very active in developing protections for patients within HMOs and publicly funded personal health services systems that are fiscally viable. States will also address access to controversial services, such as family planning. By the end of the decade, it is likely

that there will be enough momentum and shared experience at the state level to reinitiate federal-level comprehensive personal and public health care reforms. Along the way, another, more controversial, policy pathway increasingly will be taken: litigation. Following in the footsteps of the tobacco suits, there will be more court challenges to the public and personal health status quo. While this approach is provocative, in particular in redirecting accountability to industry, it will take some time to evaluate its true value, as well as to expose its weaknesses.

- *Epidemiology*. Epidemiology is the fundamental science of public health. As public health problems become more complex—both because of increased understanding of the problems and because of an increasingly integrated mix of stakeholders—public health will rely on the scientific foundation offered by epidemiology as one of its most useful guides and allies. Genetic epidemiology will help to usher in widespread genetic therapy, introducing new strategies for health promotion and disease prevention—although these strategies will not replace basic public health prevention approaches. In the area of health services evaluation, information technology will enhance epidemiological research. Constantly changing management and payment structures will make access to consistent and informative data sets difficult, however, thereby presenting major challenges to solid epidemiological evaluation of health services.

- *Universities.* Educational institutions will continue in their roles as researchers and advisors to policymakers and public health practitioners. Their role in training public health leaders will expand, especially through distance training programs and joint degree programs. Universities will also play a leadership role in studying and guiding ethical and human rights debates regarding emerging public health practices.

ENDNOTES

[1] Centers for Disease Control and Prevention. Ten great public health achievements—United States, 1900–1999. *Morbidity and Mortality Weekly Report* 1999; 48:241–243.

[2] Executive Office of the President, Office of Management and Budget, 1999.

[3] Lantz, P., et al. Socioeconomic factors, health behaviors, and mortality. *Journal of the American Medical Association* 1998; 279:1703.

[4] Centerwall, B. Race, socioeconomic status, and domestic homicide. *Journal of the American Medical Association* 1995; 273:1775.

[5] Shapiro, I., and Greenstein, R. *The Widening Income Gap*. Washington, DC: Center on Budget and Policy Priorities, 1999.

[6] Centers for Disease Control and Prevention. Measles—United States, 1997. *Morbidity and Mortality Weekly Report* 1998; 47:273–276.

[7] *Reported Tuberculosis in the United States 1997*. Atlanta, GA: Centers for Disease Control and Prevention, July 1998.

[8] Putnam, J. J., and Allshouse, J. E. Food consumption, prices, and expenditures, 1970–95. *Statistical Bulletin No. 939*. Washington, DC: Economic Research Service, U.S. Department of Agriculture, 1997.

[9] Zahodiakin, P. Methanex files intent to sue California if state bans MTBE. *Pesticide & Toxic Chemical News* 1999.

[10] Public Health Foundation. *Environmental Health Data Needs: An Action Plan for Federal Public Health Agencies*. Submitted to the Environmental Health Policy Committee Subcommittee on Data Needs. June 18, 1997.

[11] Mannino, D. M., et al. Surveillance for asthma—United States, 1960–1995. *Morbidity and Mortality Weekly Report* 1998; 47 (SS-1):1–28.

[12] Centers for Disease Control and Prevention. Forecasted state-specific estimates of self-reported asthma prevalence—United States, 1998. *Morbidity and Mortality Weekly Report* 1998; 47:1022–1025.

[13] Centers for Disease Control and Prevention. Surveillance for waterborne disease outbreaks—United States, 1993–1994. *Morbidity and Mortality Weekly Report* 1996; 45 (SS-1):1–33.

[14] Drugged waters: Does it matter that pharmaceuticals are turning up in water supplies? *Science News* (March 21) 1998; 153:187–189.

[15] Centers for Disease Control and Prevention. Incidence of foodborne illnesses. *Morbidity and Mortality Weekly Report* 1999; 48:189–194.

[16] *Occupational Employment Statistics Survey by Occupation*. Washington, DC: U.S. Department of Labor, Bureau of Labor Statistics, 1997.

[17] *Measuring Expenditures for Essential Public Health Services*. Prepared by Public Health Foundation for the Office of Disease Prevention and Health Promotion, Office of Public Health and Science, U.S. Department of Health and Human Services. November 1996, Washington D.C.

[18] *Privatization and Public Health: A Study of Initiatives and Early Lessons Learned*. Washington, DC: Public Health Foundation, September 1997. Research and writing supported by The Annie E. Casey Foundation, Baltimore, Maryland.

[19] Himmelstein, D., et al. Quality of care in investor-owned vs. not-for-profit HMOs. *Journal of the American Medical Association* 1999; 282:159–163.

CHAPTER 11

Health Behaviors

Small Steps in the Right Direction

Public health researchers in 1993 stated what public health professionals had known for a long time—that the ultimate cause of death for people in the United States is often the consequence of a combination of underlying behavioral and environmental causes.[1] Examining the top ten causes of death in the United States, those researchers illustrated the links between biomedical diseases and their underlying causes (see Table 11-1).

These classifications reveal an underlying complexity in which behavioral, social, economic, environmental, and cultural forces are inextricably related to determinants of mortality. This list of underlying causes of death can therefore be a guide to prioritizing and developing successful prevention strategies for improvement of the public's health.

To that end, it is useful to assess the trends of several of the underlying causes of death. Issues related to toxins and pollutants are discussed elsewhere in this volume as they concern environmental health (see Chapter 10). Poor diet, lack of exercise, and resultant obesity are increasingly acknowledged to be serious health risks to the individual. With widespread recognition of the health risks associated with not only primary but also secondhand tobacco smoke have come paradigm-shifting public health responses including restrictions on smoking in public and some private enterprises, landmark litigation holding industry accountable for health consequences, and restrictions on advertising.

Without refuting either the substantial effect of those behaviors on public health and society overall or the far-reaching significance of the strategic responses to them, this chapter centers attention on other behaviors associated with major public health problems. These behaviors include the abuse of alcohol, the use of illicit drugs alone and in relation to the transmission of infectious diseases, the use of firearms, and the use of tobacco as it relates to the adoption of other risk behaviors. These practices are associated with significant injury and loss to both individuals and the general public in terms of mortality and morbidity, economic consequences, and loss of personal and workforce productivity. We focus on these behaviors because we believe they represent the issues that, in the coming decade, will be the most hotly contested, mark the greatest departure from traditional understanding, and spark the greatest innovation in the coming decade.

Table 11-1. Biomedical and Underlying Causes of Death in the United States in 1990

Top Ten Biomedical Determinants

Cardiovascular disease

Cancer

Cerebrovascular disease

Chronic obstructive pulmonary disease

Unintentional injury

Pneumonia and influenza

Diabetes

HIV/AIDS

Suicide

Homicide

Top Ten Underlying Causes*

Tobacco

Poor diet

Lack of exercise

Alcohol

Infectious agents

Pollutants/Toxins

Firearms

Sexual behavior

Motor vehicles

Illicit drug use

*The original list combined poor diet and lack of exercise, for a total of nine causes.

Source: McGinnis, J. M., and Foege, W. H. Review. Actual causes of death in the United States. *Journal of the American Medical Association*, November 10, 1993; 270(18):2207–12.

ALCOHOL AND DRUG ABUSE IN AMERICA

Alcohol and drug abuse are among the most pervasive health and social problems in the United States today. In a recent survey conducted by the Gallup Organization, as many as 43 percent of adults reported having been exposed to alcoholism in their family. In addition, 45 percent of Americans reported that they, a family member, or a close friend had used illegal drugs.

Although drugs and alcohol differ in the forms of social dysfunction they wreak, they also have much in common. For example, the abuse of either increases:

- instances of unintentional injury, especially in motor vehicle crashes

- the incidence of morbidity, disability, and untimely mortality

- the danger of harm to the fetus during pregnancy

- the likelihood of engaging in unsafe sexual practices

- the spread of infectious disease—especially HIV/AIDS and hepatitis

- disruptions of family life and household roles and responsibilities

- the incidence of domestic violence, sexual assault, and suicide

- the commission of crimes, including homicide

In addition, alcohol and illicit drugs present special risks for young people, and the number of potential years of life lost to alcohol- and drug-related injuries are as significant as those lost to heart disease and cancer—the two leading causes of death in the United States.

Abuse, addiction, and their consequences appear in every socioeconomic stratum, educational level, geographic region, and ethnic and racial group. The following data are drawn from several major national studies, including the 1998 National Household Survey on Drug Abuse, and the 1998 Health Services Research Outcomes Study, and are consistent with those in several other major studies.[2]

The Scope of the Alcohol and Illicit Drug Abuse Problem in the United States

■ Overall levels have remained stable over the past 7 years, but are higher than the lowest levels ever measured.

■ Levels among youths fluctuate at high levels, but may have started to decline.

■ Youths' initiation of marijuana and cocaine are at historically high levels.

■ Males, youths, urban populations, and less educated people have the highest levels of drug use.

■ Males, urban populations, and more educated people have the highest levels of alcohol consumption.

■ Youths and young adults engage in higher levels of binge and heavy drinking.

■ The public is well aware of the problem.

Of the 218 million people in the United States age 12 and older, 52 percent were using alcohol in 1998. Of those people, about 29 percent engaged in binge drinking and 11 percent were heavy drinkers.[3] The proportion of people using alcohol in the United States has remained relatively stable overall for the past few years. In 1998, just over 6 percent of this population were using illicit drugs. That percentage constitutes 13.6 million Americans—although 78 million Americans report having tried illicit drugs at some time in their life. The total number of people using illicit drugs has remained stable since 1992, at levels roughly half the 1979 peak of 25 million users, although patterns by age category vary dramatically (see Figure 11-1).

Marijuana is the most frequently used illicit drug (see Figure 11-2). Among current drug users, 81 percent reported

marijuana use, and 21 percent of marijuana users also used other drugs. An estimated 1.8 million people—0.8 percent of the U.S. population—were current users of cocaine in 1998. That percentage has remained fairly stable over the past few years, and it represents a 68 percent decrease from the 1985 peak of 5.7 million users.

WHO IS USING AND WHO IS ABUSING?

■ *Age.* According to 1998 figures, the highest rates of illicit drug use were among young people age 16 to 17 (16 percent), 18 to 20 (20 percent), and 21 to 25 (13.5 percent). The levels then decline in successively older age groups. In contrast, more than 60 percent of people from 21 to 44 years old use alcohol, but rates of binge drinking and heavy drinking are significantly higher in the 18-to-25 age group than among older adults.

■ *Race.* Illicit drug use for African Americans (8 percent) is somewhat higher than that for whites (6 percent) and Hispanics (6 percent)—although among the young there are no differences across those racial groups. Whites have the highest rates of alcohol use (55 percent), followed by Hispanics (45 percent) and African Americans (40 percent).

■ *Gender.* Males consume higher levels of both illicit drugs and alcohol than do females (8 versus 4.5 percent for drugs, and 59 versus 45 percent for alcohol).

■ *Education.* Illicit drug use is highly correlated with educational status. Young adults who have not completed

Chapter 11: Health Behaviors

Figure 11-1. Prevalence of Illicit Drug Use by Age Cohorts (Percentage of age cohort, 1979–1997)

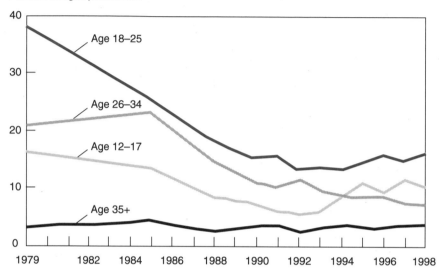

Percent using in past month

Source: Substance Abuse and Mental Health Services Association, National Household Survey on Drug Abuse, 1998.

Figure 11-2. Marijuana Is the Drug of Choice

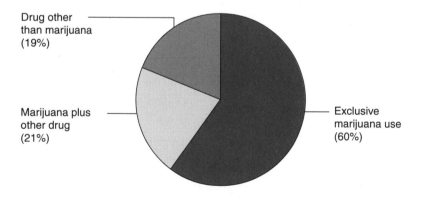

Drug other than marijuana (19%)

Marijuana plus other drug (21%)

Exclusive marijuana use (60%)

Source: Substance Abuse and Mental Health Services Association, National Household Survey on Drug Abuse, 1997.

high school have the highest rate of illicit drug use (10 percent) and college graduates have the lowest (5 percent). Conversely, the higher the level of education, the higher the proportion of people in the group who use alcohol. In 1998, 65 percent of college graduates used alcohol as compared to 40 percent of people who had not graduated from high school.

■ *Interactions.* The level of alcohol use was strongly associated with illicit drug use in 1998, as in prior years (see Figure 11-3). Within each educational level, the more a person drinks alcohol, the more likely it is that the person will also take drugs.

Concern for the Young

Alcohol use among young people has insidious consequences because youths who drink alcohol are at greater risk for the development of a serious alcohol disorder. For example, youths who initiate alcohol use when they are 15 years old are 4 times more likely to become alcohol dependent as people who start drinking at or after the age of 21 (see Figure 11-4).

Especially as it affects the young, the interaction of alcohol, drug, and tobacco use should be considered. Young smokers are 12 times more likely to also take illicit drugs and are 16 times more likely to drink alcohol heavily than are young nonsmokers. Youths who are heavy alcohol drinkers are 24 times more likely to take drugs than are young nondrinkers (see Figure 11-5).

In 1998, 19 percent of all adolescents 12 to 17 years old reported that they used

Chapter 11: Health Behaviors

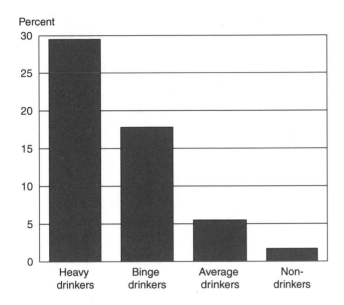

Figure 11-3. Association of Alcohol and Illicit Drug Use (Percentage of drinkers also using illicit drugs, by level of alcohol consumption)

Source: IFTF; Substance Abuse and Mental Health Services Association, National Household Survey on Drug Abuse, 1998.

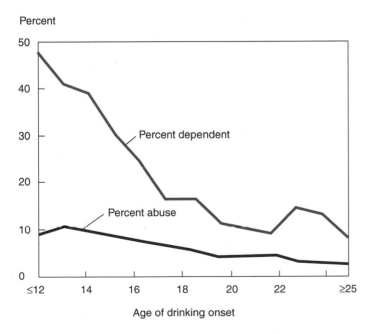

Figure 11-4. Prevalence of Lifetime Alcohol Dependency or Abuse, and Age of Drinking Onset

Source: National Institute on Alcohol Abuse and Alcoholism, Office of Policy Analysis, 1998.

alcohol. These young people are more likely to engage in binge drinking and heavy drinking. In the young adult population of 18- to 25-year-olds, levels of binge and heavy drinking have fluctuated over the past few years, but remain high.

Illicit drug use among 12- to 17-year-olds, after increasing for several years, declined slightly from 11 percent to 10 percent between 1997 and 1998. However, use of illicit drugs by young adults 18 to 25 years of age rose to its highest level, increasing to approximately 16 percent in 1998 from 14.5 percent in 1997.

Adolescents' perception of risk associated with drug use is another factor to monitor in evaluating trends in drug use. The trend in perceived risk mirrors the trend in the use of marijuana among youths. Over the years, as the perceived risk decreased, drug use increased—and vice versa (see Figure 11-6).

THE CONSEQUENCES OF SUBSTANCE ABUSE

The Toll in Injuries Caused by Substance Abuse

Injuries, both intentional and unintentional, are a major contributor to untimely death, disability, and lost productivity. The two leading causes of death from injury are motor vehicle accidents and firearms, together accounting for more than half of all injury-related deaths, and much of the time, alcohol and illicit drugs are on the scene.

Alcohol- and drug-related injuries accounted for 487,600 emergency room visits in 1996. Alcohol is a factor in

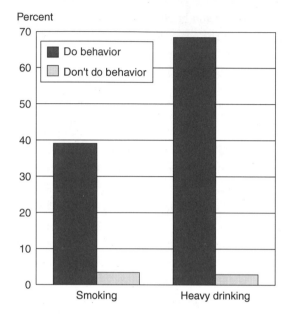

Figure 11-5. Interaction of Drugs, Tobacco, and Alcohol (Percentage of illicit drug use among youths who do and do not smoke and drink heavily)

Source: IFTF; Substance Abuse and Mental Health Services Association, National Household Survey on Drug Abuse, 1998.

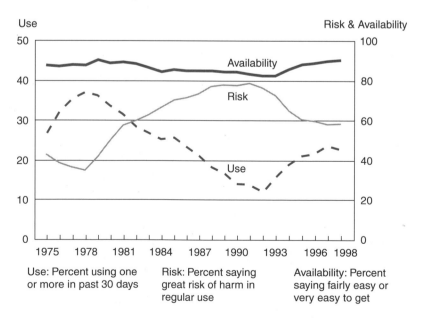

Figure 11-6. Trends in Perceptions of Availability and Risk of Regular Use, Compared with 30-Day Prevalence for Twelfth Graders

Use: Percent using one or more in past 30 days

Risk: Percent saying great risk of harm in regular use

Availability: Percent saying fairly easy or very easy to get

Source: Monitoring the Future Study, University of Michigan, 1998.

almost 60 percent of all fatal falls and, together with other drugs, figures in almost half of all fatal automobile crashes and up to 65 percent of adult drownings.[4,5] In fact, alcohol is implicated in 100,000 deaths each year, mostly from unintentional injuries, homicides, and suicides. The estimated relative risk of accidental death is 2.5 to 8 times greater among males who are heavy drinkers or alcohol dependent than among the general population.[5] Trauma victims are often found to be intoxicated, and a history of trauma is a marker for the early identification of alcohol abuse. Risk-function analysis for social consequences, which assesses the probability of occurrence of specific consequences at specified levels of alcohol consumption, associates alcohol with diminished social functioning and increased harm.

Alcohol and Drugs Causing Morbidity and Untimely Death

After smoking and obesity, substance abuse is the third leading preventable cause of mortality in the United States today. As many as 11 percent of preventable deaths in the United States are related directly to alcohol and illicit drug use. Alcohol accounts for 5 percent of premature deaths, and cirrhosis, alcoholic psychoses, and nondependent abuse of alcohol make alcohol a major contributing cause of hospitalizations.

The U.S. Department of Justice reports that 40 percent of fatal motor vehicle accidents involve alcohol. Illicit drug use is a major contributor to deaths due to overdose, suicide, homicide, motor vehicle injuries, and HIV/AIDS. Furthermore, drug-related deaths have increased 42 percent since 1990, reaching 14,218 in 1995. As Figure 11-7 shows, overall drug-related visits to the emergency room have declined slightly, but levels of heroin- and cocaine-related visits have increased.

Domestic Violence

Violent behaviors between family members causing physical and emotional harm are prevalent throughout the world. More than 1 million children in the United States are known victims of abuse and neglect, one-quarter suffering physical abuse and another quarter being sexually abused or emotionally mistreated.

Spousal and child abuse are as clearly related to alcohol abuse as are motor vehicle injuries. Alcohol and/or illicit drug use is a factor in more than 50 percent of all incidents of domestic violence. A 1993 study of more than 2,000 American couples showed that rates of domestic violence were almost 15 times higher in households where husbands were often drunk than in homes where husbands were never drunk. Alcoholism and child abuse, including incest, are tightly intertwined as well. Between 25 and 50 percent of men who commit acts of domestic violence have substance abuse problems. Not only do abusers tend to be heavy drinkers, but also the people they abuse are more likely to abuse alcohol and other drugs over the course of their lifetime. Battered women are more likely to abuse alcohol and other drugs, suffer depression, attempt suicide, and abuse their own children.[6,7,8]

Drugs, Alcohol, and Crime

Violent crimes now affect some 11 million victims annually, and drugs, alcohol, and crime go together.[9] Of the 1.7 million men and women in the nation's jails and prisons in 1997, 4 out of 10 reported using alcohol, and 6 out of 10 reported being under the influence of illicit drugs at the time of their offense. The U.S. Department of Justice reports that 40 percent of violent assaults involve the use of alcohol. Each year, 37 percent of all rapes and sexual assaults involve alcohol use by the offender, as do 15 percent of robberies, 27 percent of aggravated assaults, and nearly 25 percent of simple assaults.

Not only is substance abuse a cause of crime, it *is* a crime. More than a million arrests—over one-third of all arrests in the United States—are made each year for intoxicated driving, liquor-law violations, drunkenness, and other statutory crimes concerning alcohol and drugs. America has one of the highest incarceration rates

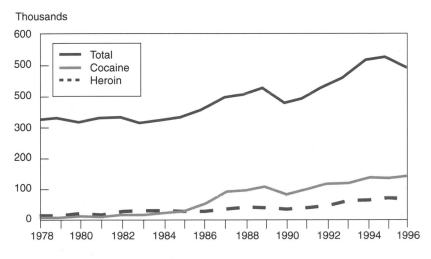

Figure 11-7. Trends in Drug-Related Emergency Room Visits, 1978–1996

Thousands

Source: Substance Abuse and Mental Health Services Administration, Health and Human Services Drug Abuse Warning Network, 1997.

Chapter 11: Health Behaviors

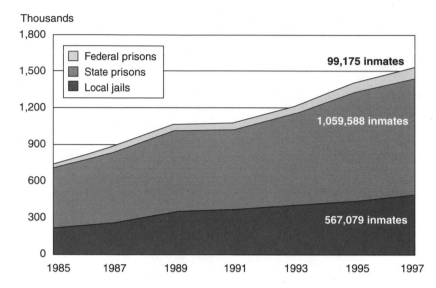

Figure 11-8. Incarcerations in Federal and State Prisons and Local Jails, 1985–1997

Thousands

Legend:
- Federal prisons
- State prisons
- Local jails

99,175 inmates

1,059,588 inmates

567,079 inmates

Source: IFTF; Substance Abuse and Mental Health Services Association, National Household Survey on Drug Abuse, 1998.

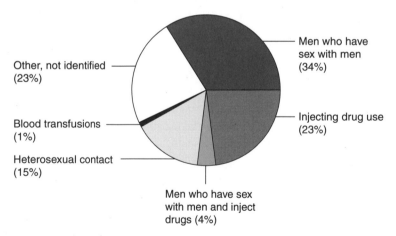

Figure 11-9. Drug Use and AIDS (Percentage of new AIDS cases by exposure category, June 1999; 46,761 total cases)

Other, not identified (23%)

Blood transfusions (1%)

Heterosexual contact (15%)

Men who have sex with men and inject drugs (4%)

Men who have sex with men (34%)

Injecting drug use (23%)

Source: Centers for Disease Control and Prevention. HIV/AIDS Surveillance Report, Mid-Year Edition, 1999.

in the industrialized world (868 per 100,000 population), and drug violations alone accounted for three-quarters of the growth in the U.S. inmate population between 1985 and 1995 (see Figure 11-8). According to FBI records of arrests from 1970 through 1997, arrests for drug abuse violations are at their highest levels ever in the United States. The number of arrests for drug abuse violations has almost doubled for adults (from 629,196 in 1985 to 1,019,621 in 1997) and have more than doubled for juveniles (from 68,122 in 1986 to 154,761 in 1997).[10]

HIV/AIDS and Sexually Transmitted Diseases

Alcohol and drug use contribute to the spread of HIV/AIDS and other sexually transmitted diseases. Impaired judgment about having sex and about condom use increases the risk of spreading an infectious disease. Behaviors associated with drug use, such as the exchange of sex for drugs and needle sharing, increase exposure to infectious diseases. More than 40 percent of AIDS cases among women are drug related. There is also evidence that alcohol and other drugs weaken the immune system, thereby increasing susceptibility to infection and disease. In fact, drug use is now the second-largest risk factor for HIV infection in the United States. As of mid-1999, approximately one-quarter of all new AIDS cases were among people using drugs by injection (see Figure 11-9).

THE COSTS

It is difficult to put a monetary value on the human suffering and loss of life associated with alcohol and other drug prob-

Figure 11-10. Economic Costs of Alcohol and Drug Abuse

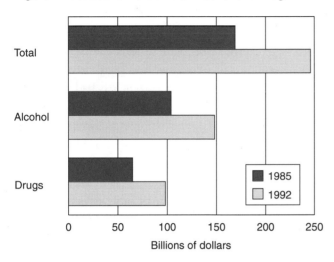

Billions of dollars

Note: Comparison reflects results of cost of illness studies.

Source: IFTF; Substance Abuse and Mental Health Services Association, National Household Survey on Drug Abuse, 1998.

the health care system, and society also feel the burden. The economic problems, which are increasing annually in absolute and proportionate terms, include:

- rising share of total health care expenditures related to alcohol and drug use

- diminished workforce productivity

- lower household incomes, in turn affecting family members

- diversion of government funds from other programs into alcohol and drug treatment

THE HEALTH CARE SYSTEM

A large part of the national health care bill is for medical expenses related to the use or abuse of alcohol, tobacco, and other drugs. Many general hospital beds are occupied by patients with alcohol-related medical conditions. When hospital admissions are related to alcohol or illicit drug use, the disorders tend to be more severe and more expensive than in other admissions. Health care costs related to substance abuse do not stop at the abuser. Children of alcoholics average 62 percent more hospital days, 24 percent more inpatient admissions, and 29 percent longer stays than do other children.

As recently reported in *Health Affairs*, national health care expenditures related to alcohol and drug abuse totaled more than $12.5 billion in 1996, with $5 billion for alcohol abuse and $7.6 billion for drug abuse. The costs of alcohol abuse are rising at an average annual growth rate of 1.7 percent, whereas the costs of drug abuse increase annually by

lems, but other, more direct costs add up to big dollars. Alcohol and other drug use is a factor in many of this country's most serious and expensive problems, including—in addition to the injuries, health risks, and crimes just described—teen pregnancy, failure at school, escalating health care costs, low worker productivity, and homelessness.

Alcohol and illicit drug abuse in the United States cost society nearly $246 billion in 1992, reflecting a 50 percent increase from 1985. Alcohol abuse accounted for 60 percent of the total and drug abuse accounted for the remaining 40 percent (see Figure 11-10).

Most of the costs are borne by the government and the individual substance abusers, although families, businesses, more than 13 percent. It is primarily the public that pays for these expenses: 63 percent ($7.9 billion) of total spending on alcohol and drug abuse came from public sources, including Medicare (13 percent), Medicaid (23 percent), other federal agencies (22 percent), and state and local agencies (41 percent).

THE WORKPLACE

Drug and alcohol abuse costs U.S. businesses more than $110 billion a year in lost workdays, accidents, and increased insurance rates. Although illicit drug users are less likely to be employed than people who do not use drugs, about 70 percent of all current adult illicit drug users and heavy drinkers are employed full time. The overall rate of current illicit drug use among full-time employ-

ees dropped from a high of 17.5 percent in 1985 to a low of 7.4 percent in 1992, and since then has remained stable.

High employment levels among drug and alcohol abusers is good news for the substance abusers, but it is bad news for the workplace. Compared to other workers, employees reporting current alcohol or drug abuse were 2 to 2.5 times more likely to have worked for three or more employers during the past year and to have skipped one or more days of work during the past month. Compared to their drug-free or alcohol-free coworkers, alcohol and drug users generally are less dependable, are less productive, have more unexcused absences, are more frequently fired, and switch jobs more often (see Figure 11-11). The abuse problem is most serious among workers in the restaurant, construction, and transportation industries.

THE POLITICS OF PROBLEMS RELATED TO ALCOHOL AND DRUG ABUSE

It is clear that alcohol- and drug-related problems are profound and seem intractable. An overview of U.S. policy efforts to reduce alcohol and drug abuse in the 20th century highlights the foundations of future directions for substance abuse politics and policies.

U.S. policies on alcohol and drugs are best understood in their historical and social context. Before Prohibition in 1933, the alcohol policy was dominated by judgments concerning an individual's behavior rather than by an understanding of alcohol abuse as both a disease and

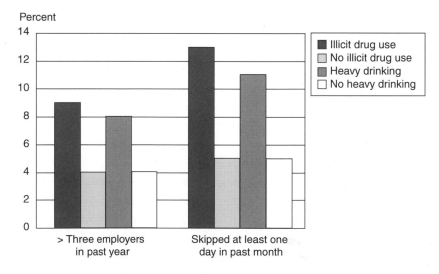

Figure 11-11. The Workplace Consequences of Drug and Alcohol Abuse: Employment History and Absenteeism

Source: IFTF; Substance Abuse and Mental Health Services Association, National Household Survey on Drug Abuse, 1998.

a social phenomenon. Prohibition's policy legacy is a supply-side approach that incorporates criminal law, drug interdiction, and incarceration more frequently than rehabilitation. Despite ever growing awareness that these Prohibition-based strategies are largely ineffective and economically unsustainable, they have been the cornerstones of national policy for more than 60 years—culminating in the national War on Drugs of the 1980s.

Accompanying this approach were arrests, fines, property forfeiture, and imprisonment for producers, sellers, and buyers. The cost to arrest, try, sentence, and incarcerate people found guilty for the more than 4 million alcohol- and other drug-related offenses committed each year is over $60 billion annually. This expenditure is a tremendous drain on U.S. resources. Incarcerating prisoners is now the most rapidly growing expense faced by governors and state legislatures.

Policy on the control of drugs and alcohol continues to be inadequate. Two particular pressures help to explain the policy impasse.

The Bifurcation of Alcohol and Drug Policy

Although both alcohol and drugs are addictive agents, U.S. policy and prevention strategies approach them quite differently, starting with the distinction in their legal status. Each has its own set of stakeholders, advocates, and opponents. Efforts to develop a comprehensive, coordinated policy are debilitated primarily by a lack of coordination between the

criminal justice system and the public health field.

The Dominance of the Criminal Justice System

From 1989 to 1997, federal spending for drug control programs increased from $6.6 billion to more than $17.1 billion, with an average annual increase of 10 percent—well above the rate of inflation. The criminal justice system has consistently received about half of these funds, whereas treatment and prevention receive a third of total funding, and other supply-side strategies and interdiction consume the remaining amount. No change to these strategic and spending priorities is in sight, as a recent House decision added $2.6 billion in law enforcement to the $17 billion already allocated for the National Drug Control Strategy.

DETERMINING THE SOLUTIONS: THE PROMISE OF PUBLIC HEALTH

Although the legacy of the War on Drugs still dominates alcohol and drug policy in the United States, there are signs of preliminary shifts in national policy. The National Drug Control Strategy of 1998 deviates from past strategies in that it attempts to approach drug control as a continuous process rather than a battle with a definitive end. It also addresses the interaction of drug, alcohol, and tobacco use. It emphasizes prevention and treatment efforts and makes a priority of tobacco and alcohol use by underage youths. The National Drug Control Strategy may finally be viewing alcohol and drug problems through a public health lens. But once the politicians and the public focus on public health, what will they see?

Ecological Approaches

The public health community has begun to shift emphasis away from individual-based strategies toward broader ecological approaches. The main goal of individual-based strategies is to increase the individual's knowledge and change his or her behavior. Although they are important, individual-based interventions are ultimately limited by the greater environment, where social drinking and experimentation are encouraged. In contrast, ecological public health strategies address alcohol and drug abuse as an interplay of individual, biological, community, family, environmental, and policy influences. For example, by working in concert, education and rehabilitation programs, peer support groups, regulation of alcohol outlets, restriction of advertising, media advocacy, and taxation can reduce alcohol and drug abuse risks for an entire community. The success or failure of an ecological approach to alcohol and drug abuse is held in the balance by several key issues that are highly controversial and unresolved. They include youth-targeted interventions, funding for treatment and rehabilitation, and the economic dynamics that shape the use and abuse of alcohol.

Youth Focus: Prevention Strategy or Politics?

With high levels of illicit drug use among 12- to 17-year-olds prevailing, and with mounting evidence that early use increases the risk of addiction, helping young people to stay away from alcohol and drug abuse is one of the most urgent issues on the substance-abuse agenda. Public sentiment supports the science. Recent survey data on American attitudes toward children's health issues show respondents citing "drugs/drug abuse" and "alcohol" among the top five serious problems facing children in America today. However, *how* to address youths' alcohol and drug use is highly controversial. Effective, environmentally based, youth-focused strategies must break through current controversy if they are to shape the future.

Demand for Treatment Is Increasing, but Who Will Pay?

Research shows that treatment not only reduces substance abuse but reduces crime as well. Criminal activity, including income-producing crimes and violent and disorderly offenses, declines by 23 to 38 percent following substance-abuse treatment. Each dollar spent on drug treatment saves Americans $7 by reducing or avoiding costs related to criminal justice, health care, and welfare activities.

Despite these findings, there is a serious gap between the need for and the provision of rehabilitation services. In 1997, 1.9 million people were enrolled in treatment programs and another 7.4 million were on waiting lists. To fulfill the potential of alcohol and drug rehabilitation, the chasm between this need and the resources available to meet it must be bridged (see Figure 11-12).

Economic Forces in Alcohol Use and Abuse

Two main factors are evolving in the understanding of economic forces in alcohol use and abuse. The first is the mount-

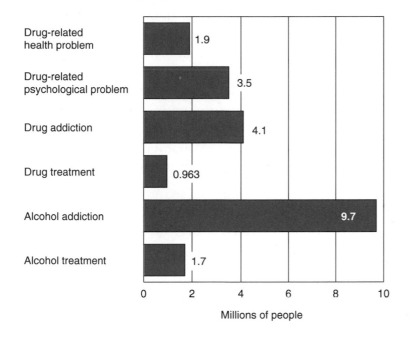

Figure 11-12. Reported Past Year Illicit Drug or Alcohol Problem Relative to Treatment (Millions of people, 1998)

Source: IFTF; Substance Abuse and Mental Health Services Association, National Household Survey on Drug Abuse, 1998.

Improving the overall quality of the social and physical environment holds the greatest promise for reducing the costs of alcohol and drug abuse in society. However, addressing these issues is inherently political, and any future advancements must shoulder the legacies of the past and the problems of today. In this context, we make the following forecasts.

- *Alcohol and drug use and health effects.* Drug use in the teenage and young adult populations will continue to be high, although recent changes in national drug policy may result in some decline. High levels will continue to be driven by marijuana use, conflicting media messages, peer pressure, risk-taking behavior, and the popular sentiment that "all use is not abuse." Alcohol and drugs will continue to be among the leading causes of morbidity, disability, and premature mortality in the United States.

- *Prevention and treatment.* The high levels of new users initiating drug and alcohol use have important implications for substance-abuse prevention efforts and treatment services. Demand for treatment will increasingly place pressure on these already strapped services. As drug-using baby boomers age, they will bring their drug-related problems with them, increasing demands on medical and Medicare services because of their large numbers and because their aging will lead to increased medical complications. Prevention efforts will increasingly target adolescents, both to protect the well-being of individuals and society and to buffer the already overburdened treatment services.

ing evidence that the public's consumption of beer, wine, and spirits is sensitive to tax, and ultimately price, increases. The second is the evidence suggesting that alcohol abuse and dependence correspond with lower earnings and income levels. The effects of economic forces differ between moderate and heavy drinkers, and strategies and conclusions must consider variations in alcohol consumption. As more sophisticated methodologies and enhanced data sets develop, approaches can increasingly shape substance-abuse prevention efforts and policy.

THE FORECAST FOR ALCOHOL AND DRUGS

Few of the problems of alcohol and drug abuse in the United States are likely to be resolved within the next 10 years.

■ *Economic and social costs.* Without radical change in policy, overall costs of alcohol and drug abuse—and their consequences in terms of such events as motor vehicle accidents and incidents involving firearms—will remain in the billions. Even with increases in prevention- and treatment-oriented efforts, the time frame for resolution of current problems is likely to exceed this 10-year forecast, especially considering that long-term consequences of alcohol and drug abuse will have a delayed impact on health care systems and government.

■ *Community-based organizations.* Expect to see more states and local communities experimenting with ecological approaches and strategies. Citizen-led initiatives will scrutinize local ordinances regarding alcohol sales and advertising, galvanizing local officials, advocates, and parents to seek out ways to reduce the influences of alcohol and drugs in their neighborhoods and to stage community events.

■ *The alcohol industry and taxation.* Despite some evidence that increased taxation of alcohol may reduce its purchase by younger and poorer people, future use of this strategy is unlikely, considering the tangled relationship between politics and industry contributions. Industry lobbying will remain strong, as evidenced by the alcohol industry's recent end to its self-imposed ban on advertising of liquor.

■ *Strategies.* Although the government will continue to place the bulk of its funding in supply-side and criminal

justice measures, prevention strategies will continue. The focus increasingly will be on ecological approaches to address the problem. Researchers will seek greater understanding of the distinctions in approaches needed for different groups such as youth, women, and heavy drinkers. Concurrently, efforts increasingly will focus on harm reduction, with mounting pressure on the government to work on suppression of consumption.

INJURY PREVENTION: A FOCUS ON GUNS

Accidents don't just happen. Injury prevention experts say that there is no physical event of a health-threatening nature that cannot be avoided or its negative consequences reduced. And yet, in the United States, unintentional injuries and violence are a major cause of death, disability, and lost productivity for people under 55. In 1995, injuries were responsible for nearly 150,000 deaths, 2.6 million hospitalizations, over 36 million visits to the emergency room, and $260 billion in societal costs.[11,12] Motor vehicle injuries, while generally declining, remain the number one injury-related cause of death. Disturbingly, what follows this largely unintentional injury-related cause of death is intentional firearm-related homicide and suicide.

Fortunately, major advances in injury prevention over the past 30 years reduced motor vehicle injury to historically low levels. Epidemiology, the core science of public health, has been a key tool in these efforts by providing the research to prevent and control injuries through legislation, environmental changes, and education. During the past 15 years, the motor vehicle traffic fatality rate has declined nearly 30 percent[13] because of developments in legislation, roadway and vehicle design, driver and pedestrian education, protective equipment, and the establishment of emergency medical services systems. Future improvements will result from the use of devices to detect and prevent driver drowsiness, vehicle-mounted sensors to warn of and avert collisions, and stricter laws governing drinking and driving

FIREARMS IN AMERICA

There are over 200 million guns in the United States.[14] Nearly 40 percent of U.S. households have at least one gun and nearly one-quarter have a handgun.[15]

These firearms are not just mounted above the hearth. Rather, many are involved in killing and injuring people: in 1997, there were 32,436 gun-related deaths in the United States—more than 88 deaths every day.[16] Indeed, rates of firearm death and injury are higher in the United States than in any other industrialized country.[17] Particularly chilling, the United States has the highest male teen homicide rate and childhood firearm death rates in the industrialized world.[18]

Solutions to firearm injury, while lying within the public health framework, also present prevention specialists with unique challenges. No other consumer product (except tobacco) remains outside the jurisdiction of a federal agency that can regulate its safety, is embroiled in constitutional and cultural controversies, and is consistently and lethally involved

in intentional injury and criminal activity. In addition, to adequately address firearm injury, public health professionals must coordinate with a complex array of fields and institutions that address criminal justice, violence, mental health, substance abuse, and poverty. These factors have required injury prevention professionals to break new ground and are catalyzing a flurry of policy, litigation, manufacturing, and advocacy actions and reactions. All told, the future of firearm injury prevention is incredibly dynamic, and its unique challenges may generate innovations useful to the broader field of injury prevention.

By 1993, firearm injuries and expenses seemed to be spiraling out of control, and the CDC estimated that by the year 2001, firearms would surpass motor vehicles as the leading cause of injury death in the United States.[13] However, levels of firearm death seem to be cyclical, and gun deaths have declined over 18 percent since 1993, with the decline occurring more in homicides and unintentional injuries than in suicides.[16] If that trend continues, within a few years firearm-related deaths could be at their lowest point since the 1950s.[19]

WHO GETS HURT

Youths, males, and minorities are the main victims of gun injuries. Men, young men in particular, are on average 6 times more likely to die by firearms than are women. African Americans are 2.5 times more likely to be killed by firearms than are whites. African American men 15 to 24 years old are nearly 5 times more likely to die by firearms than white men in that age group.[20]

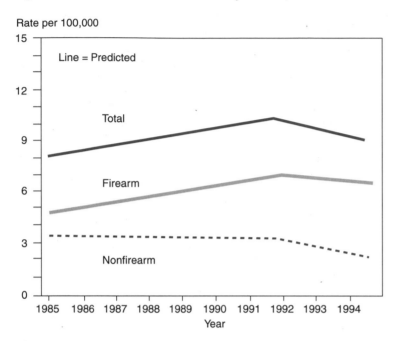

Figure 11-13. Trends in Homicide Rates by Method, 1985–1994

Rate per 100,000

Line = Predicted

Total

Firearm

Nonfirearm

Year

Note: Variance from the regression line not shown.

Source: Centers for Disease Control and Prevention. Trends in Rates of Homicide—United States, 1985–1994. *Morbidity and Mortality Weekly Report,* June 7, 1996; 45(22):460–464.

Homicides

Firearms are the weapon of choice in approximately 70 percent of U.S. homicides, and of these firearm-related deaths, 86 percent involve handguns.[21] In homes with guns, the homicide of a household member is nearly 3 times more likely than in homes without guns.[22] Youth homicide rates climbed sharply until 1994, and while consistently declining since then, remain high, especially among 15- to 19-year-olds (see Figure 11-13).

Suicides

Less recognized than homicide, suicide is a significant contributor to firearm-

related mortality. In 1997, 54 percent of all gun deaths were suicides, and 42 percent were homicides. Guns are the method of choice for nearly 60 percent of people who commit suicide.[16] In homes with guns, the risk of suicide is nearly 5 times higher than in homes without guns.[23] As with homicides, suicide rates have declined since the mid-1990s, but to a lesser degree. Suicide rates among senior adults are consistently the highest, although youth suicide is also at a historical high. Rates for African American youths have increased disproportionately, with firearms accounting for 96 percent of the increase (Figure 11-14).

Unintentional Shootings

Unintentional firearm deaths, representing only about 3 percent of all firearm-related fatalities, have been in steady decline but still firearms killed nearly a thousand people in 1998.[18] It is estimated that over 17,000 people each year are treated for unintentional, nonfatal gunshot wounds in hospital emergency departments. Unintentional shootings are also significant because they may be highly preventable, and because children are often the victims.[24]

AT WHAT PRICE?

The sticker shock of firearm injury—as measured in hospitalization, rehabilitation, and lost wages—is impressive. The cost per firearm-related fatality is higher than for any other class of fatal injury. Firearm injury also tends to generate more costly morbidity.[25] A 1999 study estimated that gunshot injuries in 1994 produced $2.3 billion in lifetime medical costs.[26] Gunshot injuries due to

Figure 11-14. Adolescent Suicide: A Black and White Comparison, 1980–1995 (Suicide rates for blacks and whites age 15 to 19, by year—United States)

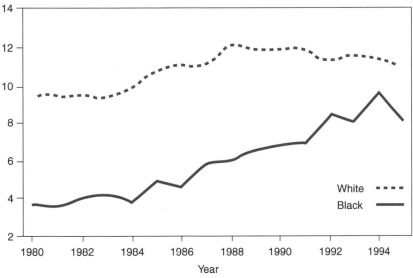

Rate per 100,000

Year

White ----
Black ——

Source: Centers for Disease Control and Prevention. Suicide Among Black Youths—United States, 1980-1995. *Morbidity and Mortality Weekly Report.* March 20, 1998; 47(10):193–106.

assaults accounted for 74 percent of total costs. Another study estimated that in 1990, total lifetime (medical and indirect) costs of firearm injuries would reach $20 billion.[27] These costs represent a huge potential liability for health care providers and payers, especially since the more serious the injury, the greater the government contribution.

FORCES DRIVING FIREARM INJURY PREVENTION

The future of firearm injury prevention will be shaped by the following factors:

- The past several years have delivered an array of prevention strategies that depart from traditional approaches

and may in fact be the building blocks of real change in the state of firearm injury in the United States.

- Overall firearm mortality is going down, with declines in homicide and unintentional shootings occurring faster than suicide. Young people, males, and minorities experience the greatest firearm injury and mortality burden. Unintentional and nonfatal firearm injuries also cause significant morbidity and mortality. If overall trends continue, gun violence will soon reach its lowest level in decades. With a wide array of interventions recently implemented, there is uncertainty as to the exact causes of the decline, making a forecast of future injury levels unstable. Each firearm injury continues to be expensive, and the associated costs are high for the public sector and for society at large.

- Surveillance and research on firearm use is increasing and will likely be a potent tool for reducing gun use in crime and for understanding the nature of firearm injuries and prevention strategies. However, much more needs to be done before surveillance can be considered truly comprehensive throughout the country.

- A significant number of firearm experts suggest that that debate has reached an impasse on issues such as the Second Amendment right to bear arms or the risks and benefits of gun ownership.[28] Instead, they call for a focus on policy that regulates guns as consumer products, restricts gun ownership based on criminal history, and curtails illegal gun commerce. With broad public support (see Table 11-2), these strategies may shape the prevention framework for the coming decade.

■ Firearm regulation tends to lack adequate comprehensiveness and coordination at the federal level, with some important exceptions. Most change in gun policy is originating from state-level activity, but is characterized by great variability: some state regulations strengthen firearm control, while others may weaken firearm injury prevention. Most local regulatory action continues to be limited by state pre-emption laws and public-private business arrangements.

■ Efforts to reduce firearm injuries are increasingly focused on the distribution and manufacture of firearms, in particular on regulation of handguns as consumer products and reduction of the illegal sale of guns. While some controversy exists concerning specific strategies, evidence is mounting that regulations such as licensing and registration laws, background checks, and purchasing limits can be effective in limiting the distribution of firearms and in decreasing their involvement in crime. At the same time, there is still no federal regulatory agency to provide consumer product oversight and the lethality of guns and ammunition is increasing.

■ Lawsuits are increasingly common. Similar to the reframing of guns as consumer products, litigation attempting to hold manufacturers and sellers responsible for the damage their products cause is on the rise. Hoping to imitate the success of tobacco litigation, these suits argue that firearm manufacturers can design and market their products in ways that are less likely to cause death and injury. While the success and implications are uncertain, the reward could be great and the plaintiffs are lining up to sue.

THE FORECAST FOR FIREARMS

Current firearm injury prevention policy will require time to reach its full effect, making precise levels of associated changes in firearm injury uncertain within the 10-year time frame of our forecast. However, a growing body of

Table 11-2. Support Among National Poll Respondents for Policies to Regulate Firearms

Policy	Percent who favored or strongly favored prohibition	
	All Respondents	Respondents who owned guns
Regulation of guns as consumer products		
Childproofing	88	80
Personalization	71	59
Magazine safeties	82	75
Loaded chamber indicators	73	60
Prohibition of gun purchases for people convicted of crimes		
Violence or illegal use of firearm	83–95	70–91
Alcohol or drug abuse	71–92	59–89
Reduction of the illegal sale of guns		
Tamper-resistant serial numbers	90	85
One-gun-per-month	81	53
Mandatory handgun registration	82	72

Source: IFTF; Teret, S. P. et. al. Support for new policies to regulate firearms. *New England Journal of Medicine.* 1998; 339(12):813–18.

evidence on the effectiveness of and support for innovative firearm injury prevention strategies makes it likely that improvements in the field will be pronounced in a longer-term, 20- to 30-year, scenario.

The network of surveillance systems across the country is developing, facilitating rigorous evaluation of new prevention programs and policies. Investment in the power of information will shape debate and reduce controversy, ultimately having a major impact on future policy and program development.

Guns will be scrutinized more often by policymakers as "consumer products" and increasing legislative pressure will attempt to control their manufacture and design. While the National Rifle Association will resist these efforts, it is likely that the more fiscally vulnerable manufacturing industry will be receptive to adopting certain standards. However, unless firearms are brought under the purview of a federal consumer product regulatory agency, progress toward safer guns will be slow.

In parallel, the public will gradually unwrap the gun from the American flag, change focus from the final user of firearms to the manufacturer and distributor, and increasingly identify with firearms as consumer products. Increased grassroots organization of victims, such as the Bell Campaign (using the Mothers Against Drunk Driving model), physicians, and police organizations will lead the way, along with increased participation by foundations. This rise in focused community activism, grounded in growing knowledge of which interventions work, may build the bridge between broad public support for reductions in firearm injury and social action.

Lawsuits against the gun industry will continue to increase. The impact of these suits will not be felt immediately and the long-term consequences are uncertain, even if the plaintiffs are successful. For example, it is possible that many gun manufacturers will go bankrupt in the course of these proceedings, which could ironically consolidate gun manufacturer power.

TOBACCO USE AND HEALTH

From decades of research on tobacco use and its negative effects on health, tobacco has been identified as the single greatest preventable contributor to disease and premature death in the nation—greater than illicit use of drugs, motor vehicle accidents, firearms, toxic agents, microbial agents, and alcohol combined.[29] It kills more than 400,000 Americans each year and causes heart disease; cancers of the lung, larynx, mouth, esophagus, and bladder; and chronic lung disease. Approximately $50 billion of total medical costs each year are directly attributable to tobacco use.[30]

Over the past 25 years, significant progress has been made in the health and medical fields documenting the adverse health effects of tobacco use and their related costs. The body of scientific knowledge about tobacco use and its effects on human health is massive and incontrovertible. A causal relationship exists between cigarette smoking and disease; further, nonsmokers also incur serious health problems from environmental tobacco smoke (ETS) or second-hand smoke. Use of smokeless tobacco causes a number of serious oral health problems, including cancer of the mouth, periodontitis, and tooth loss. Cigar use causes cancers of the larynx, mouth, esophagus, and lung. Today, tobacco use is the leading preventable cause of morbidity and premature mortality in the United States.

HISTORICAL OVERVIEW

In the past, helping people quit smoking was the primary focus of efforts to reduce tobacco use. This strategy has been a critical one, since smoking cessation at all ages reduces the risk of premature death. In recent years, however, the focus of tobacco control has expanded to include strategies to prevent kids from starting to smoke, limit exposure to ETS, and stop minors' access to tobacco products.

Efforts to prevent individuals from starting to smoke center on controlling youth access to tobacco products because approximately 90 percent of all initiation of tobacco use occurs among persons 18 years of age or younger.[31] Initiation of smoking at younger ages is associated with a longer duration of smoking and an increased likelihood of nicotine dependence.[31] The decision to use tobacco is nearly always made in the teenage years and about one-half of young people who take up smoking continue to use tobacco products as adults. Therefore, communities have begun taking steps to restrict youth access. Some policies include stepping up enforcement of existing laws, restricting tobacco advertising and licensing, and increasing penalties for selling to minors.

The past two decades have also seen greater recognition of the health hazards resulting from exposure to ETS. ETS is a combination of smoke exhaled by the smoker and the smoke that comes from the burning end of a cigarette, cigar, or pipe. The U.S. Environmental Protection Agency concluded in January 1993 that ETS kills an estimated 3,000 adult non-smokers from lung cancer each year.[32] What's more, nonsmokers exposed to ETS have higher death rates from cardiovascular disease than unexposed non-smokers.[33] To help control the effects of ETS, workplaces have begun shifting to smoke-free environments, as have restaurants and bars.

The Tobacco Settlement

On November 16, 1998, the attorneys general of eight states and the nation's four major tobacco companies agreed to settle more than 40 pending lawsuits brought by states against the tobacco industry.

Many supporters of the settlement nationwide worked to ensure that settlement funds were earmarked for health and health care purposes. Unfortunately, in many states this effort was unsuccessful. Instead of creating health-focused tobacco settlement trust funds, many of the first payments are being placed into general funds or going to other social programs. Many believe this outcome to be a huge loss that reflects, in part, the lack of political clout of members of the tobacco control community at large.

TODAY'S CHALLENGES

Racial/Ethnic Disparities

Although lung cancer incidence and death rates vary widely among racial/ethnic groups, lung cancer is the leading cause of cancer death for African Americans, Hispanics, Asian Americans/Pacific Islanders, and Native Americans as well as whites, with rates of tobacco-related cancers high among African American men.[34] Furthermore, it has been observed that immigrant populations, especially Southeast Asian male immigrants, have high rates of smoking that may buoy the smoking rates among racial/ethnic groups.

Nationally, cigarette-smoking prevalence increased in the 1990s among African American and Hispanic adolescents after several years of substantial decline among these adolescents. Educational attainment accounts for only some of the difference in smoking behaviors. Declines in smoking prevalence were greater among African American, Hispanic, and white men who were high school graduates than among those with less formal education.[34] Further, members of racial/ethnic groups are less likely than the general population to participate in smoking cessation groups and to receive cessation advice from health care providers.[34] Research suggests that barriers may include limited cultural competence of health care providers and a lack of transportation, money, and access to health care. Other social and cultural factors are likely to further account for these differences.

Smoking Prevalence Rates Among Children Age 12 to 13 Are Increasing

The continued financial strength of the tobacco industry relies on youth initiation and uptake of smoking as adult smokers either quit or die. The average young smoker begins at age 14.5 and is a daily smoker by age 18. Unfortunately, data indicate that the industry has been successful in reaching its goal. An interesting finding in these data concerns smoking among 12- to 17-year-olds in ethnic communities. Despite the data cited above indicating high rates of smoking prevalence among adult African Americans and Native Americans, in 1997 youths of color experienced lower smoking prevalence rates than whites, with a striking difference of 9 percentage points between white youths (12.5 percent) and African American youths (3.6 percent).[34]

Smokers Are Not Uniformly Counseled to Quit by Health Care Providers

Although smokers cite a physician's advice to quit as an important motivator for cessation, physicians and other health care clinicians, such as dentists, often fail to assess smoking status and even to advise smokers to quit. It is estimated that more than 70 million people are currently enrolled in some type of managed health care plan. Despite the managed care industry's stated interest in prevention, an alarming 68 percent of smokers report getting no help from their doctor or health insurance plan to stop smoking (see Figure 11-15).

Since 1997, national guidelines have been available from the Agency for Health Care Policy and Research regarding smoking cessation. All major health care agencies and associations recommend routine tobacco use cessation counseling for adults and adolescents who smoke.

Chapter 11: Health Behaviors   181

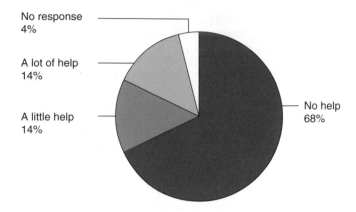

Figure 11-15. Few Smokers Report Getting Help to Quit Smoking (Responses to the question: How much help did you get from your doctor or health insurance plan in the past 12 months to try to quit smoking?)

No response 4%

A lot of help 14%

A little help 14%

No help 68%

Source: *California Managed Health Care Improvement Task Force Survey of Public Perceptions and Experiences with Health Insurance Coverage,* UC Berkeley and Field Research Corporation, 1997.

THE IMPACT OF NOT COUNSELING SMOKERS TO QUIT ON PREGNANT WOMEN, THEIR FAMILIES, CHILDREN, AND UNBORN CHILDREN

Women who smoke during pregnancy are more likely to have the following: pregnancy complications, premature birth, stillbirth, and babies with low birth weight, a leading cause of infant mortality.[35] Further, it has been shown that prenatal smoking and ETS compromise the fetal and neonate immune system, thereby leaving a newborn more susceptible to infectious disease.[36] There is also significant evidence that a dose-response relationship exists between prenatal smoking and the incidence of Sudden Infant Death Syndrome (SIDS). ETS exposure in young children has been found to be a significant risk factor for several acute upper and lower respiratory tract illnesses such as bronchitis and

pneumonia, chronic middle ear infections, and greater rates of asthma.

LACK OF STRONG, UNITED LEADERSHIP AMONG TOBACCO CONTROL STAKEHOLDERS TO DESIGN AN EFFECTIVE STRATEGY TO OUTFOX THE TOBACCO INDUSTRY

Throughout communities in America, tobacco control forces are mobilized to counter the tobacco industry. Historically the tobacco control forces in many states have been guilty of infighting that has weakened their effectiveness. And the size of the "force" is small. On the heels of losing the battle to use the tobacco settlement dollars for health, there is a clear need for statewide leadership and replenished resources.

The new leadership could assist in reframing the tobacco control issue to one of population health improvement—highlighting the role of tobacco use in statewide rates of morbidity and mortality. Greater efforts could be made to educate the public and policymakers about effective strategies to decrease tobacco use. For example, coverage of nicotine replacement therapies by health plans is limited, despite the evidence of their role in assuring smoking cessation. Further, many believe that the war against the tobacco industry is over—noting the absence of smoking in public places and the decline of smoking rates from 1955 to 1990.

THE FUTURE OF TOBACCO

The challenges that exist in tobacco control today are legion. Investments in any or all of the areas above could lead to improved health and productivity for many Americans. In addition to these issues, consideration should be given to the following areas:

- *Continue to strengthen local and statewide policy development to prevent tobacco use.* In communities across America, the tobacco industry is making considerable progress in introducing the public, especially young adults, to its products. Tobacco control experts point to problems with continued use of signage in storefronts, sponsorships, and promotions. Of particular concern is bar promotions in which ads are placed in entertainment newspapers to bring young adults to bars where cigarette samples are distributed. Also, on college campuses, students are being recruited to set up parties at which cigarettes are distributed. These are examples of local practices that could be addressed through enforcement of existing laws as well as the adoption of new policies.

- *Support community and statewide efforts to prioritize use of tobacco settlement funds for health and health care programs.* Although efforts to use the tobacco settlement to fund health and health care programs have failed in many states, initial plans are under way in some states to urge the legislatures to reconsider the issue next year. The outcome of this policy change would improve the health of large numbers of people. To achieve this goal, tobacco control stakeholders will need assistance with strategic planning and public education activities, as well as an infusion of new leadership.

WILD CARDS

ALCOHOL AND DRUGS

- Medical technologies, particularly rational drug design, ignite a tidal wave of drug abuse as a new generation of "designer" drugs that bind to specific mood receptors in the brain enter the illegal drug market.

- The alcohol industry follows the tobacco industry—up in smoke. Public opinion turns against the alcohol industries with growing organization of nondrinkers' rights groups.

- A deep economic recession leads to a further loss of access to emergency care that will follow the accompanying erosion of the large municipal hospitals that care for major injuries.

INJURY PREVENTION

- Kids organize a Stop the Pain Campaign, striking a moral chord with the public that even politicians can't resist—comprehensive federal gun control legislation is passed.

- A long economic recession sets in across America: unemployment, crime, and gun violence rise to unprecedented levels.

- A wave of new high-tech weapons, such as laser weapons and polymer guns, hits the streets. Government and emergency systems are not prepared, so initially high injury rates result.

- The United Nations and the WHO create a treaty restricting small arms trade. All but the United States ratify the treaty, resulting in international sanctions against the United States until the gun industry is stopped.

TOBACCO

- The public supports increased taxes on cigarettes. Congress passes a hefty per pack tax that cuts youths' consumption of cigarettes in half.

- The FDA regulates tobacco as a drug. Smoking rates, especially among youths, decline to unprecedented levels.

- The public becomes apathetic about the health consequences of smoking, the media become bored with the smoking issue, the tobacco control movement fragments, and nothing more is done to change smoking behaviors.

ENDNOTES

1 McGinnis, J. M., and Foege, W. H. Review. Actual causes of death in the United States. *Journal of the American Medical Association.* November 10, 1993; 270(18):2207–12.

2 The 1998 National Household Survey on Drug Abuse. National Institute on Drug Abuse, National Institute on Alcohol Abuse and Alcoholism. *The Economic Costs of Alcohol and Drug Abuse on the United States, 1992.* The Lewin Group. *The 1998 Health Services Research Outcomes Study.* Office of Applied Studies of the Substance Abuse and Mental Health Services Administration. *The Ninth Special Report to the U.S. Congress on Alcohol and Health.* Secretary of Health and Human Services, U.S. Department of Health and Human Services, Public Health Service, National Institute of Health, National Institute on Alcohol Abuse and Alcoholism, June 1997.

3 The National Household Survey on Drug Abuse defines current alcohol or illicit drug use as consumption at least once in the past month; binge drinking as five or more drinks on the same occasion at least once in the past month; and heavy drinking as five or more drinks on the same occasion at least 5 different days in the past month. Results from the study include people living in households and in some group quarters, such as dormitories and homeless shelters.

4 FARS, National Highway Traffic Safety Administration, 1993 and 1994.

5 Eighth Special Report to the U.S. Congress on Alcohol and Health, National Institute on Alcohol Abuse and Alcoholism, 1993.

6 Collins, J. J., and Messerschmidt, M. A. Epidemology of alcohol-related violence. *Alcohol Health and Research World.* 17(2):93–100.

7 U.S. Department of Health and Human Services, National Institute on Alcohol Abuse and Alcoholism, 1993.

8 Widom, C. S. *Child Abuse and Alcohol Use.* Research Monograph 24: Alcohol and Interpersonal Violence: Fostering Multidiscipli-nary Perspectives. Rockville, MD: National Institute on Alcohol Abuse and Alcoholism, 1993.

9 U.S. Department of Justice, Bureau of Justice Statistics, Crime in the United States, Washington, DC.

10 *Sourcebook of Criminal Justice Statistics.* 25th ed. K. Maguire and A. Pastore, eds. Baton Rouge, LA: Justice Department, Office of Justice Programs, Bureau of Justice Statistics, Claitors Publishing Division, December 1998.

11 National Vital Statistics System, National Center for Health Statistics, CDC; Johns Hopkins Center for Injury Research and Policy.

12 Bonnie, R. J., Fulco C. E., and Liverman C. T., eds. *Reducing the Burden of Injury, Advancing Prevention and Treatment.* Committee on Injury Prevention and Control, Division of Health Promotion and Disease Prevention. Institute of Medicine. Washington DC: National Academy Press, 1999.

13 Centers for Disease Control and Prevention. Deaths resulting from firearm- and motor-vehicle-related injuries—United States, 1968–1991. *Morbidity and Mortality Weekly Report.* January 28, 1994; 43(3).

14 Guns in America: National Survey on Private Ownership and Use of Firearms, by Philip J. Cook and Jens Ludwig. National Institute of Justice, Research in Brief. May 1997. U.S. Department of Justice. NCJ 165476.

15 Johns Hopkins Center for Gun Policy and Research, National Opinion Research Center. *Fall 1998 National Gun Policy Survey: Questionnaire with Unweighted Frequencies and Weighted Percentages.* Baltimore, MD: The Johns Hopkins Center for Gun Policy and Research, 1999.

16 Hoyert, D. L., Kochanek, K. D., and Murphy, S. L. Deaths: final data for 1997. *National Vital Statistics Reports.* 1999; 47(19).

17 Krug, E. G., et al. Firearm-related deaths in the United States and 35 other high- and upper-middle-income countries. *International*

Journal of Epidemiology. April 1998; 27(2):214–21.

18 Centers for Disease Control and Prevention. Rates of homicide, suicide and firearm-related death among children—26 industrialized countries. *Morbidity and Mortality Weekly Report.* February 7, 1997; 46(5).

19 Wintemute, G. J. The future of firearm violence prevention: building on success. *Journal of the American Medical Association.* August 4, 1999; 282(5):475–78.

20 *National Vital Statistics Reports.* June 30, 1999; 47(19).

21 Federal Bureau of Investigation. *Uniform Crime Reports for the United States: 1997.* Washington, DC: U.S. Department of Justice, 1998.

22 Kellermann, A. L., et al. Gun ownership as a risk factor for homicide in the home. *New England Journal of Medicine.* 1993; 329:1084–91.

23 Kellermann, A. L., et al. Suicide in the home in relation to gun ownership. *New England Journal of Medicine.* 1992; 327:467–72.

24 Sinauer, N., Annest, J. L., and Mercy, J. A. Unintentional, nonfatal firearm-related injuries. *Journal of the American Medical Association.* 1996; 275:1740–43.

25 Miller, T. R., and Cohen, M. A. Costs. In *The Textbook of Penetrating Trauma.* R. R. Ivatury and C. G. Cayten, eds. New York: Williams & Wilkins, 1996.

26 Cook, P. J., et al. The medical costs of gunshot injuries in the United States. *Journal of the American Medical Association.* August 4, 1999; 282(5):447–54.

27 Max, W., et al. Shooting in the dark: estimating the cost of firearm injuries. *Health Affairs.* Winter 1993; 12(4):171–85.

28 Teret, S. P., et al. Support for new policies to regulate firearms. Results of two national surveys. *New England Journal of Medicine.* September 17, 1998; 339(12):813–8.

29 Centers for Disease Control and Prevention, Office on Smoking and Health/ National Center for Chronic Disease Prevention and Health Promotion. Adult Tobacco Use in California: Health Impact and Cost 1997.

30 Smoking Cessation: Clinical Practice Guideline No. 18. Agency for Health Care Policy and Research, U.S. Department of Health and Human Services, Rockville, MD, 1996, p. 5.

31 Gemson, D. H., et al. Laying down the law: reducing illegal tobacco sales to minors in central Harlem. *American Journal of Public Health.* 1998; 88:936–39.

32 Making Your Workplace Smoke-Free: A Decision Maker's Guide. U.S. Department of Health and Human Services, and Center for Disease Control and Prevention, Office of Smoking and Health, 1996, p. 2.

33 Steenland, K., et al. Environmental tobacco smoke and coronary heart disease in the American Cancer Society CPS-II cohort. *Circulation.* 1996; 94:622–28.

34 U.S. Department of Health and Human Services. *Tobacco Use Among U.S. Racial/ Ethnic Minority Groups—African Americans, American Indians and Alaska Natives, Asian Americans and Pacific Islanders, and Hispanics: A Report of the Surgeon General.* Atlanta, GA: U.S. Department of Health and Human Services, Centers for Disease Control and Prevention, National Center for Chronic Disease Prevention and Health Promotion, Office on Smoking and Health, 1998.

35 DiFranza, J. R., and Lew, R. A. Morbidity and mortality in children associated with the use of tobacco products by other people. *Pediatrics.* 1996; 4:560–68.

36 Castellazzi, A. M., et al. Effect of active and passive smoking during pregnancy on natural killer-cell activity in infants. *Journal of Allergy and Clinical Immunology.* 1999; 103(1):172–73.

CHAPTER 12

Expanded Perspective on Health

Beyond the Curative Model

As we move into the new millennium, we're broadening our perspective on health. Until recently, biomedical understanding of disease and the definition of health as "the absence of disease" provided the fundamental framework in which modern medicine evolved and the curative model of medical care predominated. The curative model narrowly focuses on the goal of cure; that is, the eradication of the cause of an illness or disease. Although cure is unquestionably an appropriate goal, other goals are important as well: restoring functional capacity; relieving suffering; preventing illness, injury, and untimely death; promoting health; and caring for those who cannot be cured.

Cure-oriented medicine reveres the "hard" medical sciences, and it ignores behavioral phenomena that are not entirely explained by biological science. Effective cure is presumed to be contingent on diagnosis gained from knowledge of disordered function. Treatment is supposed to be derived from empirical research on clinical outcomes. In fact, on careful analysis, a significant component of medical practice is neither knowledge based nor supported by evidence.

The cure-oriented approach to medicine and health is highly invested in a bio-medical perspective that values scientifically based data over other information and accepts evidence-based approaches to treatment over those less rigorously derived. The curative model has created a hierarchical structure of relationships among health professionals: physicians who command the most biomedical knowledge also command the most authority. Our society has granted this authority to physicians and has entrusted them with the role of granting or denying the legitimacy of matters related to health and disease. Thus, indirectly, the medical profession has defined health in the narrow meaning of disease according to a curative biomedical model.

In the past quarter century, the record of biomedical discovery and progress has been spectacular, and yet on critical analysis our ability to diagnose and treat disease has had no more than a modest impact on the public's health. Despite improved diagnostic and therapeutic capabilities and an unprecedented expenditure of resources, we are not the most healthy of peoples among the developed nations. Perhaps an obsession with disease has unintentionally relegated health to a position of secondary importance. The health care delivery system is still organized, staffed, and financed on the assumption that its central task is to use biomedical interventions to provide care for people facing acute episodes of illness.

From many quarters comes evidence that our view of health should be expanded to encompass mental, social, and spiritual well-being. An expanded view of health integrates the concepts of curative medicine (absence of disease) with public health (absence of excessive mortality, morbidity, and risk factors for disease), and adds productive functioning and well-being. This expanded view of health recognizes the importance of mental factors, social support, income, and behavior in avoiding disease and disability. The expanded view of health moves beyond attention only on disease to incorporate the concept of *salutogenesis,* the generation and maintenance of health.[1]

The American public expects accurate and timely diagnosis and treatment of illness and disease, but this same public has new expectations for avoiding illness and disease and wants more attention directed to chronic diseases, aging, and terminal care at the end of life. The public's understanding of health and its interest in healthy lifestyles have advanced remarkably in the past decade. As individuals, each of us wants to be healthy and fully functional. To achieve this, we must adopt an expanded view of health that adds, to physical health, essential mental, social, and spiritual components. This expanded definition of health has three implications:

■ For individuals to function at their best, health as defined here is a necessary precondition.

■ Impairment of any component of health can predispose to or cause disease and create an unhealthy state.

■ Mental, social, and spiritual factors, singly and collectively, influence behavior and therefore health.

An expanded view of health assumes a particular meaning for the elderly, age 65 years or older, who currently constitute 13 percent of the population. Less concerned about life span than about life quality during the remaining life span, this cohort embraces all elements of health with the same tenacity of younger generations. Evidence shows that maximum human life span is fixed and that improvements in health can affect only mean life span and not maximum attainable life span. Nonetheless, all adult generations want to postpone the effects of aging and to avoid or mitigate age-related disabilities. Concern about aging thus becomes a largely unarticulated part of the equation for health, and it requires special consideration as we develop a much broader concept of what health and being healthy means to all segments of the population.

Because socioeconomic status is a powerful determinant of health and disease, recognizing and understanding the relevance of an expanded definition of health to the lower socioeconomic segments of the population will be critical to improving the collective health of the nation. Improving the health of the middle- and upper-income segments of the population is important, but it is clearly insufficient if achieving substantial improvement in our national health status is the goal.

Finally, who can and will integrate an expanded view of health into the planning and delivery of health care, and what should be the roles of government, providers, employers, and consumers in advocating changes that recognize and respect this new definition of health? This multifaceted question will be addressed in a later section of this chapter, but posing the question at this point may heighten sensitivity to the issue.

DEFINITION OF HEALTH

A definition of health must have equal applicability to everyone: to the fully well; to those who are unwell because of disease or illness that is treatable or even curable and for whom the goal is a return to health; and to that growing segment of the population with genetic or acquired impairment, such as those with chronic disease or disability. Furthermore, the definition of health must at the same time represent an objective to be attained and a yardstick by which to judge the state of health. Health can be applied to an individual, a community, or a nation, and in each instance the goal is to be as healthy as possible within constraints that cannot be changed.

Perfect or ideal health is a state of complete physical, mental, social, and spiritual well-being. For the vast majority of our population, being healthy means functioning as fully as possible under present circumstances. Health is a composite of interdependent components that, even if less than perfect, are optimal for the individual. As it is used in an expanded definition of health, each of the four components of health is a necessary contributor. Neglect of any component

of health predisposes one to, or creates, an unhealthy state. Although this may seem to be stating the obvious, the concept is critical to understanding the significance of an expanded view of health and the factors that determine it.

CONTRIBUTORS AND DETERMINANTS OF HEALTH

■ *Physical.* In the traditional meaning of health and disease, disease represented disordered form and function whereas health was the absence of disease. Physical health and well-being is essential to good health but taken alone is insufficient. Physical health incorporates functional as well as structural integrity. Impairment of function in the biomedical view of disease is assumed to have an organic basis. "Functional" is used in another way that may be confusing because in clinical practice "functional" describes a set of symptoms that have no organic basis. Thus, in medical practice, a "functional" illness is one that has no known physical (organic) causes and is assumed to reflect mental factors.

■ *Mental.* Mental factors include more than the absence of mental illness. They extend to emotional states (e.g., depressed feelings short of clinical depression), dispositions (e.g., hostility, optimism), and beliefs and expectations (e.g., self-esteem, self-control, self-efficacy). Mental factors, such as stress, depression, and inability to change lifelong habits, contribute to the onset of some disorders, the progression of many, and the management of all. Understanding the role of mental factors in health and disease may be the most important contribution of an expanded view of health.

- *Social.* This term has two different meanings in relation to health. Social position or status refers to the tiered structure of society and the activity of its members. This meaning of "social" cannot be dissected neatly from the more descriptive use of socioeconomic status. The position of an individual, a family, or a community in the social order is an ordering of employment, income, wealth, education, voice, and health status. In this context, the multiple social and economic factors that influence health are central not only to the development of disease but also to its treatment and outcome.

  The other meaning of "social," and the one implied in using "social well-being" in the expanded view of health, relates to relationships rather than to social order. This is the term "social" as reflected in "sociable," and refers to companionship, enjoying the company and support of family and friends, and often having intimate and supportive relationships with one or more individuals or groups. The social interaction often takes place in a community of people in the same or a similar socioeconomic stratum.

  A recent body of research has focused on the role of social networks in maintaining individual health. Social networks build communities and contribute to social capital. Social engagement and social support, regardless of an individual's socioeconomic status, are basic human needs

without which a person cannot be fully healthy. Evidence clearly shows the powerful influence of social support on recovery from myocardial infarction and breast cancer.

- *Spiritual.* Spirit is the thinking, motivating, and feeling part of humankind and involves a code of ethics and philosophy. Spirituality usually, but not necessarily, involves belief in a higher power. A spiritual person has a set of beliefs that give meaning to life, and for many this belief provides a basis for faith and trust in an otherwise disorderly and unfeeling world. A growing body of evidence supports religious involvement as an epidemiologically significant protective factor that promotes healthy behavior and lifestyles. When shared in a community, it also provides social support, which buffers stress and enhances coping mechanisms. The consistency and robustness of studies involving the role of spirituality in health have led to the emergence of a growing area of research called the "epidemiology of religion." That spiritual factors promote good health, aid in recovery from illness, and contribute to the state of well-being that characterizes health has generated growing support: the questions are how and why? The mental, social, and spiritual components of health may have distinctive but similar salutary effects mediated through psychoneuroendocrine pathways.[2]

STRESS

Stress is unavoidable, and although the socioeconomically disadvantaged may have fewer means and mechanisms for coping with stress and are thus more vulnerable to it, all of us are exposed to stress on an almost daily basis. Some amount of stress is part of life and is both natural and normal, but when stress is sustained and unrelieved it has deleterious effects on the function of endocrine and immune systems, lowering resistance and increasing vulnerability to illness, disease, and accelerated aging. This mechanistic explanation has garnered scientific support, although any claim for thoroughly understanding this complex series of interactions is premature.

Research is under way to examine how the biological consequences of adaptations to stress interact with other factors and what impact this has on health. Nancy Adler and Bruce McEwen, among others, have promoted the concept of an allostatic (adaptive) system that includes stress-induced activation of the hypothalamic-pituitary-adrenal axis, the autonomic nervous system, the cardiovascular system, the metabolic systems, and the immune system.[3] Allostatic response systems are coupled closely with an individual's psychological makeup, prior experience, and available resources for coping with stress. Stress turns on an allostatic response, and as long as the response is time limited, protection dominates over adverse consequences. However, weeks or years of repeated exposure to elevated levels of stress can result in allostatic load, with resultant damaging physiological consequences. Allostatic load can result from frequent stress, from inability to shut off responses when stress is terminated (a feature of aging), or from inadequate allostatic responses. Inability to control their lives and the daily stresses

on people in lower socioeconomic groups lead to allostatic load, sustained allostatic responses, and a downward spiral toward poor health, illness, and untimely death.

SOCIOECONOMIC STATUS AS A DETERMINANT OF HEALTH

Whether social class is measured by income, education, employment grade, or prestige, it determines the resources that are available to meet life's challenges and thereby influences the control that one has in shaping life. In 1980, the publication of the *Black Report* showed the statistical association between illness and social class in England and Wales. Physical and mental health, the statistics showed, ran parallel to social rank. With the introduction of universal health care through the National Health Service in the United Kingdom, these differences in health status among different socioeconomic groups were not reduced but actually became greater! This observation provided early evidence that the availability of universal health care does not eliminate the root cause of lower health status among the socioeconomically disadvantaged. In England, commoners die sooner than aristocrats, sergeants have more heart attacks than generals, office clerks are more depressed and anxious than office managers. In America, the lower middle class is more mortal, morbid, symptomatic, and disabled than the upper middle class. With each step down the educational, occupational, and income ladders comes an increased risk of health-related symptoms, illness, chronic disease, and early death.

Socioeconomic status (SES) exhibits a linear relationship to the incidence of illness and avoidable death. Universal health insurance would have an imperceptible effect on reducing the socially driven inequalities in health: SES differences in health are evident in countries with universal coverage; differences can be shown between levels at the upper range of the SES hierarchy; and SES differences appear in a wide range of diseases, some of which are treatable and others that are not.

Cross-national studies have shown the importance of the size of the gap between the wealthy and the less well off. In any given society, the greater the gap in income between the rich and the poor, the lower is the average life expectancy. This consistent observation explains why a country as wealthy as the United States, which spends more money per capita on health care than any nation in the world but has an ever-widening gap between rich and poor, endures an average life expectancy that is conspicuously low among the developed nations.[5]

Research into health and illness has now recognized the contribution of social, economic, and environmental factors to health, and a critical body of evidence is beginning to document the influence of these factors on morbidity and mortality.[6] However, the fact that a group of determinants—social isolation, social class, and depression—predict health outcomes across *all* diseases has been largely ignored in mainstream medical research on disease. Recognizing shared determinants of health rather than only those unique to specific diseases will enrich and modify our understanding of how internal and external factors interact to produce health or lead to illness and disease. Recognition and acceptance of the seminal role of upstream determinants of disease by the medical establishment, policymakers, and funding sources can create a virtual transformation in our approach to creating healthier individuals, communities, and nations.

WHAT'S NEW? WHY NOW?

The answer to "What's new?" is straightforward: dependence on a biomedical model to define disease and health has been rendered insufficient by a growing body of evidence that health involves much more than freedom from active disease or illness and that upstream environmental and psychosocial determinants of disease deserve parity with conventional biological theories. The answer to "Why now?" is more complex, but the reasons revolve around three factors. First, an increasingly empowered public expects more than our existing system of health care provides. When individuals become ill or impaired by

"Alternative," "Holistic," "Expanded": What's in a Name?

The search for a label that adequately captures the essential concepts embedded in an expanded view of health has been a colossal failure. No single word or phrase seems to capture what it means to view health and disease through a wider lens, to define health as a state that moves outside of a biomedical model, and to realize that upstream determinants of disease go beyond genetic endowment and access to care to even more critical socioeconomic, behavioral, social, and environmental factors. Labels in the contemporary lexicon, such as "mind-body" and "holistic," have connotations of their own and further fail the test of descriptive accuracy.

"Alternative medicine," "integrative medicine," and "complementary medicine" merit similar objections as labels, although these descriptors contain elements that pass the test of compatibility with an expanded view of health. The public's acceptance and use of alternative or complementary medical practices must be interpreted as an indication that these alternative providers fulfill some unmet need. Interestingly, much of "alternative" medicine is practiced in a way similar to biomedicine but using different forms of intervention and treatment—for instance, using herbs instead of prescription drugs.

Concluding that no single term or phrase could satisfy the goal, we decided to follow the lead of the Center for the Advancement of Health and use the descriptive label of "an expanded view of health," leaving an open field for creative lexicographers. An expanded view of health maintains and extends beyond the biomedical model. An expanded view of health applies not only to individuals but also to communities and even nations; and each component in an expanded view of health has been validated by evidence submitted to scientific scrutiny. It is the evidence-based foundation of an expanded view of health that makes it such a powerful summons to rethink and then redirect our approach to health, illness, and healing.

chronic disease or aging and seek medical care, they want a healing relationship with clinicians. Second, unless corrective measures are implemented very soon, a growing segment of our population, spanning all socioeconomic classes but most severely affecting those at the bottom, will be exposed to avoidable illness and disease and excessive mortality. Third, the nation's bill for health care and health-related disability will continue to rise until an expanded view of health promotes maintenance of

full health, greater attention to the management of chronic diseases, and elimination of upstream determinants of diseases that are determined by socioeconomic status.

A coincidental factor is the new dominance of managed care organizations. Managed care is organized to function according to the fundamental precepts of public health, health promotion, epidemiology, and population-based medicine. Assuming responsibility for the health of a defined population, as capitated managed care organizations do, creates a compelling incentive to improve and maintain the population's health. An expanded view of health is the formulation of the desired goal—good health—for a population as well as for each of its members. An expanded view of health also requires an understanding of upstream determinants of health and illness, which in turn provides insight into the roles of socioeconomic factors, behavior, and social capital. An expanded view of health was no less relevant to the practice of medicine in the era preceding managed care than it is today, but the public's changed expectations of physicians and managed care's new focus on health maintenance and disease prevention have made it appear so.

CONSUMER EXPECTATIONS

Led by health-conscious seniors and a generation of baby boomers who seem to view aging as an option subject to free choice, the medical establishment is confronting a mandate to move beyond the curative model to become engaged in

Evidence-Based Studies: What the Research Shows

Psychological and social factors—how we think, feel, and behave—profoundly influence the onset of some diseases, the progression of many, and the management of nearly all.

- In a large study covering 13 years, depressed and socially isolated persons were four times more likely to have a heart attack than those who were not depressed or isolated.[7]

- A 7-year follow-up of women diagnosed with breast cancer showed that those who confided in at least one person in the 3 months after surgery had a 7-year survival rate of 72.4 percent, as compared to 56.3 percent for those who didn't have a confidant.[8]

- In another study, women with advanced breast cancer who attended weekly therapy groups survived an average of 18 months longer than women who did not get such support. Four years later, one-third of the support group attendees were still alive whereas all of the non-attendees had died.[9]

- In a study examining the correlation of social ties to susceptibility to common cold viruses, increased diversity in types of ties to friends, family, work, and community was significantly associated with increased host resistance to infection.[10]

- In a study examining 232 elderly patients who had elective open heart surgery, those who did not participate in any group and did not receive strength and comfort from religion had three times the risk of dying as those who lacked one or the other.[11]

preserving health and preventing illness and disease. The public believes that medicine has overpromised cure as the be-all and end-all. Preventive maintenance, after all, is standard procedure for other industries. Although the enlightened consumer wants to be healthier and understands the importance of maintaining good health, a quick-fix mentality still encounters difficulty in understanding the hard work of health. Today's physicians were taught nothing about changing their patients' behavior, and with only on-the-job experience as a source of knowledge, most physicians falter when confronted with the conse-

quences of their patients' unhealthy behavior, such as obesity, tobacco use, and sexually transmitted disease. A medical curriculum reconfigured by an expanded view of health would require a course in behavioral psychology.

Their needs unmet in biomedicine, millions of Americans flock to practitioners of alternative medicine in growing numbers. Medical practitioners should not become providers of alternative medicine, and vice versa. Unlike any time in the past, the medical establishment will be more open to adopting an expanded view of health and enlarging the scope of medical practice—not with the intention of introducing alternative methodologies but rather with the goal of providing more comprehensive medical care to patients. Does this mean that for the first time your own physician may ask you about your own social support, spiritual practices, and allostatic load? Quite possibly.

DETERIORATING HEALTH CONDITIONS

The issue most urgently in need of resolution is the deteriorating health status of a growing segment of our population. To argue that this is a socioeconomic problem caused by macroeconomic forces and erosion of social capital, and not a matter of health, indicates a failure to recognize their connectedness and interdependence. In fact, separation of socioeconomic status and health is artificial, and this basic tenet is embedded in an expanded view of health. The emerging reality is that a growing segment of the population in the world's richest nation is unhealthy despite a per capita expenditure on health care that is the largest among developed countries. Health status declines with socioeconomic status, amidst a dizzying array of alarming observations: use of illicit drugs, alcohol, and tobacco by a generation of young people growing up in an environment without social order and support and one in which risky behavior is *de rigueur;* a growing population of underinsured and uninsured, many of whom lack financial resources for access to basic health care as the health care safety net unravels; a rapidly expanding population of the elderly with significant health needs, such as preventive services, social support, and the treatment of depression; and at all levels of society, avoidable illness and disease attributable to ignorance, unhealthy behavior, lack of education, and disintegration of family structure and social support.

Certain mental, social, and spiritual matters fall directly into an expanded scope of health care and can be dealt with by a physician or other health professional without outside intervention. Other socioeconomically driven health concerns cannot be resolved by the health professions, and by their nature these issues will require major shifts in political and social policy and cooperation from other professions for significant change to occur. When the medical profession adopts an expanded view of health, as it almost certainly will, it acknowledges the direct relevance of upstream determinants of health and disease that have received little or no attention because of the profession's historical focus on a biomedical model of disease.

Quite apart from concern about distributive equity, why should the higher-income classes become concerned about poor health conditions among the less advantaged? The reasons are as follows:

- The cost of preventable illness and disease is enormous and is increasing due to premature births, teenage pregnancies, AIDS, avoidable hospitalizations, communicable diseases, and the consequences of substance abuse and other risky behaviors. To the direct cost of providing health care must be added the indirect costs of lost productivity and chronic disability as a consequence of poor health.

- Communicable diseases are a major public health concern that is amplified by the worldwide emergence of drug-resistant infectious agents, involving not only common infections like *E. coli* and *Staphylococci* but less common infections, such as tuberculosis, HIV, and even plague. Any reservoir of disease constitutes a direct threat to all Americans because we share the same air, water, food, space, and transportation—and even needles and medical devices. We ignore the problem at our own peril.

GLOBAL HEALTH PERSPECTIVE

As we enter the next century, cardiovascular disease, depression, and injury-related death and disability will be major health-related concerns.[12] An individual's behavior and allostatic response to life's stresses create a profile of risk factors for developing and dying from cardiovascular disease. Risk-promoting behaviors—smoking, alcohol abuse, sedentary lifestyle, and unhealthy eating habits—have a dominant role in the evolution of cardiovascular disease, and stress-related factors promote disease progression and affect recovery from acute events such as myocardial infarction. Social and mental factors often contribute to the course of cardiovascular disease, either in promoting its progression or in favoring full recovery from an acute episode of clinical illness.

Depressive illness and risk-taking behaviors are subjects that have been largely excluded from consideration in a traditional biomedical model of disease. Depressive illness—clinically significant but falling short of disabling major depression—affects a surprisingly large proportion of the elderly population, and among the nonelderly, including adolescents, depression directly or indirectly causes poor health. An expanded view of health recognizes depressive illness as a cause of disability to be as legitimate as diabetes, asthma, and peptic ulcer. Because depressive illness looms so large as a major health concern, the rapid adoption of an expanded view of health that addresses its cause and treatment becomes a matter of high priority.

Injury-related death and disability involves the innocent as well as the guilty, the cautious as well as the careless, the abuser as well as the abused. The emergency room log in any major hospital records the consequences of traffic accidents, industrial injuries, personal assaults, alcohol- and drug-related accidents and criminal behavior, in-home injuries, and spousal abuse. The myriad factors in this melange of misery have social, cultural, mental, behavioral, racial, environmental, occupational, economic, and circumstantial elements that with few exceptions have been considered outside the scope of medical education and practice. A study of intentional and accidental injuries inevitably exposes the major role that socioeconomic status plays in causing injury, either directly or indirectly. Social, mental, and spiritual health is incompatible with the risky, antisocial, and violent behavior that often leads to serious injuries and their consequences. The prevention of injuries and injury-related morbidity and mortality, formerly considered the responsibility of public health officials, must become a legitimate concern of medicine and other health professions.

The Wild Card

In predicting global health concerns in the next century, great uncertainty surrounds the threat posed by drug-resistant infections. Particularly at risk of contracting drug-resistant infections are people in the lowest socioeconomic groups, the homeless, those with chronic diseases or in poor general health, stressed adults in all socioeconomic strata, prisoners, and the depressed and malnourished elderly. Rapid and remarkable advances in biotechnology, molecular genomics, and structure-based drug design are expected to prevent regional outbreaks and global epidemics of these potentially fatal and contagious drug-resistant diseases. Furthermore, there is deep concern regarding the existence of biologic weapons in the hands of terrorists, based on the difficulty of defending against biologic weapons attacks and the lack of a rapid and effective response system. One can imagine the global spread of an infectious agent, which overwhelms the health system's capacity and takes countless lives worldwide. This threat is being taken seriously because the risk of a biologic global disaster is a frightening possibility.

THE FUTURE: SHIFTING PARADIGMS

Thomas Kuhn pointed out that scientific advances come in the form of paradigm shifts only when existing conceptual models break down and are no longer able to explain observable facts.[13] New paradigms will emerge in the next century by expanding the definition of health. An expanded view of health is the engine that will drive the paradigmatic shifts shown in Table 12-1.

The first shift is from rigid adherence to the biomedical model to an expanded, multifactorial view of health. While the scientific model looks only at biological indicators of health, the expanded model goes beyond this to include social, mental, and spiritual, as well as physical, health. This shift in focus will lead to the regular provision of psychosocial and other services that are not currently in the health care mainstream. How the medical community acts to encourage

the shift will greatly affect the speed and degree to which it happens.

A second shift will be from attention solely on acute episodic illness to the management of chronic illness. This shift is already beginning in the treatment of certain populations, such as patients with end-stage renal disease, diabetes, and asthma. Chronic disease management programs have evolved rapidly because they provide better care at lower cost across the health care continuum. Protocols, case managers, prevention strategies, and the coordination of ancillary services have proven the value of chronic disease management by reducing the frequency and severity of acute illness episodes. In increasing numbers, health plans and large medical groups are forming their own teams to manage populations of chronically ill patients or "carving out" their care to multispecialty networks that assume full responsibility for all patient care needs on a per capita basis.

The shift in focus from individuals to groups reflects several factors. In the traditional model, a physician–patient relationship implied a contract in which physicians vowed to do everything for their patients that might be of possible benefit even if the benefit had marginal value. The terms of this contract recognized no financial restraints, and in a FFS system of care the cost was not a major consideration. As managed care has evolved over the past decade, the principles of population-based health care, already being practiced in the public health system, are beginning to be exploited and adopted by the private sector.

Table 12-1. Paradigm Shifts

Biomedical	Expanded View
Rigid adherence to the biomedical model	→ Expansion to incorporate a multifactorial view of health
Attention solely to acute episodic illness	→ Chronic illness management
Focus on individuals	→ Focus on communities and other defined populations
Cure as uncompromised goal	→ Adjustment and adaptation to disease for which there is no cure
Focus on disease	→ Focus on diseased person *and* the disease

Source: IFTF.

Community-centered health care is population-based medicine as it applies to defined groups of people. As in public health, the central theme is using finite resources to achieve the best health outcome for the entire population. The importance that an expanded view of health assigns to the maintenance of health and prevention of disease fits perfectly into a public health–population-based model of health and health care.

Cure-oriented medicine recognized a cure as the objective and measure of success, and it used diagnosis and treatment as the means of obtaining it. Palliation—lessening the severity of disease without curing it—was viewed as a compromise and deserving of less interest and attention. Many chronic diseases, such as asthma, diabetes, cardiovascular disease, and multiple sclerosis, and the conditions that accompany the aging process are by their nature incurable. An expanded view of health care promotes individual adjustment and adaptation to live with these conditions comfortably. However, the functionality and quality of life for those afflicted can be immeasurably improved by using available palliative measures. The aging of our population and the longer survival of patients with chronic diseases will shift greater attention to the health benefits of palliative interventions.

The final shifting paradigm moves from an exclusive focus on the disease to a broader focus on the importance of the person bearing the disease. The diseased person not only has an illness with organic manifestations but is also an individual with unique and relevant social, mental, and spiritual characteristics. Also, many chronically ill patients suffer from multiple comorbid conditions, and the focus on one disease could subordinate the impact of something equally debilitating. Restoration of the patient's health requires elimination of the disease if that is possible, but in addition it requires that attention be directed to the patient's mental, social, and spiritual well-being in keeping with an expanded view of health.

THE PARADIGM SHIFT: EVOLUTION OR REVOLUTION?

Amid signs that the shift is under way, it is sobering to be reminded that institutionalized values and processes change slowly, and that change may not follow a direct linear progression from "what was" to "what will be." To be sure, consumers who want a more personalized relationship with health professionals have spoken, and this message will result in a less formal and more symmetrical physician–patient interchange. However, this manifestation of change may be more cosmetic than fundamental.

With little doubt, by the year 2005, the impact of an expanded view of health will be recognizable although neither dramatic nor widespread. Physicians will be reluctant change makers because the generations of physicians in the current workforce learned, believe in, and practice according to the biomedical, bipolar view of disease and health. Interviews with practicing physicians provide ample evidence that medicine's disdain for soft science—and in their view the psychosocial sciences are soft—is alive and well. In time, many will be converted to proponents of an expanded view of health, but inroads by 2005 will be modest. Economic rewards for attention directed toward social, mental, and spiritual well-being do not exist in current reimbursement guidelines. However, by 2005, the principles underlying an expanded view of health will become general knowledge. This knowledge, reinforced by evidence that health and recovery from disease are profoundly affected by social, mental, and spiritual factors, may create a momentum that could accelerate the paradigm shift in the years following. Unless political forecasts are mistaken, by 2005, no significant legislation will be enacted that will remedy socioeconomic inequities. Health plans may expand mental health benefits in response to consumer pressure, but the impact of this change will be limited.

By 2010, the new physicians entering practice will have been educated in a different school of thought, and this new generation will understand an expanded view of health. They will need no convincing to practice accordingly, if the practice environment permits. They will augment a growing number of older colleagues in advocating major restructuring of programs to correct socioeconomic ills. The year 2010 will see the beginning of major government initiatives by legislators who understand the interconnectedness of socioeconomic status, the public's health, and the nation's productivity. At the most fundamental level, legislators will have the political will to invest in community-level programs because, for the first time in our history, they can justify the expenditure of public funds for programs that fully benefit the nation's health, productivity, and economic welfare.

This forecast may seem overly optimistic. For certain, change will be incremental and geographically uneven. Although 2010 will look different from 2005, we do not expect major change to occur until the middle of the following decade. It will be an evolution rather than a revolution, the progress of which will be painfully slow unless and until the medical establishment openly adopts an expanded view of health. It will need to bring the full force of its professional position to bear in declaring that mental, social, and spiritual factors are legitimate components of health. Physician-led advocacy is a necessary prerequisite for meaningful change in the way that consumers, providers, employers, health plans, governments, and legislators think about health and its immediate determinants. We bet on physicians to get the ball rolling, but predicting when is a matter of pure speculation.

WILD CARDS

- A major economic recession could postpone crucial legislation and governmental programs and at the same time expand the socioeconomically disadvantaged segment of the population.

- An educated public, a groundswell of community involvement, and a critical number of federal and state legislators with the political will to provide financial support for programs that provide educational opportunities, training for skilled jobs, health care including mental health care, and public health services that focus on behavioral modification could drive the pace of change at a more rapid rate than we forecast.

Chapter 12: Expanded Perspective on Health   199

ENDNOTES

[1] McKinley, J.B. *Preparation for Aging.* Keikkinen, E., et al. (eds.) New York: Plenum Press, 1995.

[2] Kiecolt-Glaser, J.K. Psychoneuroimmunology and health consequences. *Psychosomatic Medicine* 1995; 57:269–274.

[3] McEwen, B.S. Hormones as regulators of brain development. *Acta Paediatrica* 1997; 422:41–44.

[4] Taira, D.A., et al. The relationship between patient income and physician discussion of health risk behaviors. *Journal of the American Medical Association* 1997; 278:1412–17.

[5] Adler, N., et al. Socioeconomic inequalities in health. *Journal of the American Medical Association* 1993; 269:3140–45; Wilkinson, R.G. Income distribution and life expectancy. *British Medical Journal* 1992; 304:165–68.

[6] Gruman, J. Introduction for superhighways for disease. *Psychosomatic Medicine* 1995; 57:207.

[7] Pratt, L.A., et al. Depression, psychotropic medication, and risk of myocardial infarction. *Circulation* 1996; 94:3123–29.

[8] Maunsell, E., Brisson, J., and Deschenes, L. Social support and survival among women with breast cancer. *Cancer* 1995; 76:631–637.

[9] Spiegel, D., et al. Effect of psychosocial treatment on survival of patients with metastatic breast cancer. *Lancet* 1989; 2:888–890.

[10] Cohen, S., et al. Social ties and susceptibility to the common cold. *Journal of the American Medical Association* 1996; 277:1940-44.

[11] Oxman, T.E., Freeman, D.H., and Manheimer, E.D. Lack of social participation or religious strength and comfort as risk factors for death after cardiac surgery in the elderly. *Psychosomatic Medicine* 1996; 57:5–15.

[12] *The Global Burden of Disease.* Murray, C.J.L, and Lopez, A.D. (eds.). Cambridge, MA: Harvard University Press, 1996.

[13] Kuhn, T. *The Structure of Scientific Revolutions*, 3rd ed. Chicago: University of Chicago Press, 1996.

Chapter 12: Expanded Perspective on Health

Glossary

Listed below are brief explanations of common health care terms used in this forecast. Many of these glossary terms and resource citations are taken from the Public Health and Health Care Administration Glossary of Terms Web page of the University of Washington (http://weber.u.washington.edu/~hserv/hsic/resource/glossary.html).

ACADEMIC MEDICAL CENTER (AMC)

A group of related institutions including a teaching hospital or hospitals, a medical school and its affiliated faculty practice plan, and other health professional schools.

ADJUSTED AVERAGE PER CAPITA COST (AAPCC)

A county-level estimate of the average cost incurred by Medicare for each beneficiary in the FFS system. Adjustments are made so that the AAPCC represents the level of spending that would occur if each county contained the same mix of beneficiaries. Medicare pays health plans 95 percent of the AAPCC, adjusted for the characteristics of the enrollees in each plan. See also Medicare Risk Contract.

AID TO FAMILIES WITH DEPENDENT CHILDREN (AFDC) PROGRAM

A federally financed program for single-parent families, designed to provide welfare for single parents who cannot, without assistance, take proper care of their children.

AMBULATORY CARE

Medical services provided on an outpatient (nonhospital) basis. Services may include diagnosis, treatment, surgery, and rehabilitation.

BENEFIT PACKAGE

Services covered by a health insurance plan and the financial terms of such coverage, including cost sharing and limitations on amounts of services.

CAPITATION

A method of paying health care providers or insurers in which a fixed amount is paid per enrollee to cover a defined set of services over a specified period, regardless of actual services provided.

CASE MANAGEMENT

Monitoring and coordinating the delivery of health services for individual patients to enhance care and manage costs; often used for patients with specific diagnoses or who require high-cost or extensive health care services.

Case Mix

The mix of patients treated within a particular institutional setting, such as the hospital. Patient classification systems like DRGs can be used to measure the hospital case mix.

Copayment

A fixed amount of money paid by a health care plan enrollee (beneficiary) at the time of service. The health plan pays the remainder of the charge directly to the provider. This is a method of cost sharing between the enrollee and the plan and serves as an incentive for the enrollee to use health care resources wisely.

Deductible

The amount of money an insured person must pay "at the front end" before the insurer will pay. The reason for introducing this concept into health care coverage is primarily to discourage unnecessary use of services, and also to reduce insurance premiums, as all claims have a minimum amount that the insurer will be spared on every claim.

Diagnosis-Related Group (DRG)

A hospital patient classification system developed at Yale University. The current payment system for Medicare is based on the federal government's setting a predetermined price for the "package of care" in the hospital (exclusive of physician's fees) required for each DRG. If the hospital can provide the care for less than the DRG price, it can keep the difference; if the care costs the hospital more than the price, the hospital has to absorb the difference. Originally each DRG was intended to contain patients who were roughly the same kind of patient in a medical sense and who spent about the same amount of time in the hospital. The groupings were subsequently redefined so that, in addition to medical similarity, resource consumption was approximately the same within a given group.

Direct Contracting

Direct contracting usually refers to a service (e.g., substance abuse treatment) that an employer contracts directly to save money on its employees' health plan, leaving employees free to choose among other eligible providers for their primary, obstetric, pediatric, and other medical care needs.

Disproportionate Share Hospital (DSH)

A Medicare term for a hospital serving a higher than average proportion of low-income patients.

Enrollee

A person who is covered by health insurance.

ERISA

The Employee Retirement Income Security Act. ERISA exempts self-insured health plans from state laws governing health insurance, including contribution to risk pools, prohibitions against disease discrimination, and other state health reforms.

FEE-FOR-SERVICE (FFS)

A method of paying the provider whatever fee he or she charges on completion of a specific service.

GATEKEEPER

The person responsible for determining the services to be provided to a patient and coordinating the provision of the appropriate care. The purposes of the gatekeeper's function are (1) to improve the quality of care by considering the whole patient, that is, all the patient's problems and other relevant factors; (2) to ensure that all necessary care is obtained; and (3) to reduce unnecessary care and cost. When, as is often the case, the gatekeeper is a physician, she or he is a primary care physician and usually must, except in an emergency, give the first level of care to the patient before the patient is permitted to be seen by a specialist

GRADUATE MEDICAL EDUCATION (GME)

The period of medical training that follows graduation from medical school, commonly referred to as internship, residency, and fellowship training.

GROSS DOMESTIC PRODUCT (GDP)

The total current market value of all goods and services produced domestically during a given period; differs from the gross national product by excluding net income that residents earn abroad.

GROUP-MODEL HMO

An HMO that pays a medical group a negotiated, per capita rate, which the group distributes among its physicians, often under a salaried arrangement.

HEALTH CARE PROVIDER

An individual or institution that provides direct medical services (e.g., physician, hospital, laboratory). This term should not be confused with an insurance company, which "provides" insurance.

HEALTH PLAN EMPLOYER DATA AND INFORMATION SET (HEDIS)

A set of standardized measures of health plan performance. HEDIS permits comparisons between plans on quality, access and patient satisfaction, membership and utilization, financial information, and health plan management.

HEALTH INSURANCE

Insurance that covers the patient for health care, including physician and hospital services.

HEALTH INSURANCE PURCHASING COOPERATIVE (HIPC)

A local board created under managed competition to enroll individuals, collect and distribute premiums, and enforce the rules that manage the competition.

Health Maintenance Organization (HMO)

A managed care plan that integrates financing and delivery of a comprehensive set of health care services to an enrolled population. HMOs may contract with, directly employ, or own participating health care providers. Enrollees are usually required to choose from among these providers and, in return, have limited copayments. Providers may be paid through capitation, salary, per diem, or prenegotiated FFS rates.

Health Plan

An organization that acts as an insurer for an enrolled population.

Independent Practice Association (IPA)

An HMO that contracts with individual physicians or small physician groups to provide services to HMO enrollees at a negotiated per capita or FFS rate. Physicians maintain their own offices and can contract with other HMOs and see other FFS patients.

Managed Care

Any system of health payment or delivery arrangements where the plan attempts to control or coordinate use of health services by its enrolled members in order to contain health expenditures, improve quality, or both. Arrangements often involve a defined delivery system of providers with some form of contractual arrangement with the plan.

Medicaid

A state/federal health benefit program for the poor who are aged, blind, disabled, or members of families with dependent children. Each state sets its own eligibility standards.

Medical Loss Ratio

The ratio of benefits paid out to premiums collected for a particular type of insurance policy. Low loss ratios indicate that a small proportion of premium dollars were paid out in benefits, while high loss ratios indicate that a high percentage of the premium dollars were paid out as benefits.

Medical Savings Account (MSA)

A health insurance option consisting of a high-deductible insurance policy and a tax-advantaged savings account. Individuals would pay for their own health care up to the annual deductible by withdrawing from the savings account or paying out of pocket. The insurance policy would pay for most or all costs of covered services once the deductible is met.

Medicare

The federal health benefit program for the elderly and disabled that covers 35 million Americans or about 14 percent of the population for an annual cost of over $120 billion.

MEDICARE RISK CONTRACT

A contract between Medicare and a health plan under which the plan receives monthly capitated payments to provide Medicare-covered services for enrollees and thereby assumes insurance risk for those enrollees. A plan is eligible for a risk contract if it is a federally qualified HMO or a competitive medical plan.

MEDIGAP INSURANCE

Privately purchased individual or group health insurance policies designed to supplement Medicare coverage. Benefits may include payment of Medicare deductibles and coinsurance and balance bills, as well as payment for services not covered by Medicare. Medigap insurance must conform to one of ten federally standardized benefit packages.

MORBIDITY

A measure of disease incidence or prevalence in a given population, location, or other grouping of interest.

MORTALITY

A measure of deaths in a given population, location, or other grouping of interest.

NATIONAL HEALTH EXPENDITURES (NHE)

Total spending on health services, prescription and over-the-counter drugs and products, nursing home care, insurance costs, public health spending, and health research and construction.

NETWORK-MODEL HMO

An HMO that contracts with several different medical groups, often at a capitated rate. Groups may use different methods to pay their physicians.

OUT-OF-POCKET EXPENSE

Payments made by an individual for medical services. These may include direct payments to providers as well as payments for deductibles and coinsurance for covered services, for services not covered by the plan, for provider charges in excess of the plan's limits, and for enrollee premium payments.

OUTCOME

The result of a medical intervention on a patient.

PART A MEDICARE

Medical Hospital Insurance (HI) under Part A of Title XVIII of the Social Security Act, which covers beneficiaries for inpatient hospital, home health, hospice, and limited SNF services. Beneficiaries are responsible for deductibles and copayments.

PART B MEDICARE

Medicare Supplementary Medical Insurance (SMI) under Part B of Title XVII of the Social Security Act, which covers Medicare beneficiaries for physician services, medical supplies, and other outpatient treatment. Beneficiaries are responsible for monthly premiums, copayments, deductibles, and balance billing.

Partial Capitation

An insurance arrangement where the payment made to a health plan is a combination of a capitated premium and payment based on actual use of services; the proportions specified for these components determine the insurance risk faced by the plan.

Per Diem Payments

Fixed daily payments that do not vary with the level of services used by the patient. This method generally is used to pay institutional providers, such as hospitals and nursing facilities.

Personal Health Care Expenditures

These are outlays for goods and services related directly to patient care.

Point-of-Service (POS) Plan

A health plan with a network of providers whose services are available to enrollees at a lower cost than the services of nonnetwork providers. POS enrollees must receive authorization from a primary care physician in order to use network services. POS plans typically do not pay for out-of-network referrals for primary care services.

Practice Guideline

An explicit statement of what is known and believed about the benefits, risks, and costs of particular courses of medical action, intended to assist decisions by practitioners, patients, and others about appropriate health care for specific clinical conditions.

Preferred Provider Organization (PPO)

A health plan with a network of providers whose services are available to enrollees at lower cost than the services of nonnetwork providers. PPO enrollees may self-refer to any network provider at any time.

Prepaid Group Practice Plan

A plan in which specified health services are rendered by participating physicians to an enrolled group of persons, with a fixed periodic payment made in advance by or on behalf of each person or family. An HMO is an example of a prepaid group practice plan.

Primary Care

Primary care is the provision of integrated, accessible health care services by clinicians who are accountable for addressing a large majority of personal health care needs, developing a sustained partnership with patients, and practicing in the context of family and community.

Primary Care Case Management (PCCM)

A Medicaid managed care program in which an eligible individual may use services only with authorization from his or her assigned primary care provider. That provider is responsible for locating, coordinating, and monitoring all primary and other medical services for enrollees.

PROSPECTIVE PAYMENT

A method of paying health care providers in which rates are established in advance. Providers are paid these rates regardless of the costs they actually incur.

PUBLIC HEALTH

Activities that society does collectively to ensure conditions in which people can be healthy. This includes organized community efforts to prevent, identify, preempt, and counter threats to the public's health.

RELATIVE VALUE SCALE (RVS)

An index that assigns weights to each medical service. The weights represent the relative amount to be paid for each service. The RVS used in the development of the Medicare Fee Schedule consists of three cost components: physician work, practice expense, and malpractice expense.

RESOURCE-BASED RELATIVE VALUE SCALE (RBRVS)

A relative value scale that is based on the resources involved in providing a service.

RISK ADJUSTMENT

Increases or reductions in the amount of payment made to a health plan on behalf of a group of enrollees to compensate for health care expenditures that are expected to be higher or lower than average.

RISK SELECTION

Enrollment choices made by health plans or enrollees on the basis of perceived risk relative to the premium to be paid.

SINGLE-SPECIALTY GROUP PRACTICE

Physicians in the same specialty pool their expenses, income, and offices.

SKILLED NURSING FACILITY (SNF)

An institution that has a transfer agreement with one or more hospitals, provides primarily inpatient skilled nursing care and rehabilitative services, and meets other specific certification requirements.

SOLO PRACTICE

A physician who practices alone or with others but does not pool income or expenses.

STAFF-MODEL HMO

An HMO in which physicians practice solely as employees of the HMO and usually are paid a salary.

SUPPLEMENTAL INSURANCE

Any private health insurance plan held by a Medicare beneficiary, including Medigap policies and postretirement health benefits.

SUPPLEMENTAL MEDICAL INSURANCE (SMI)

The part of Medicare through which persons entitled to Part A Medicare, the Hospital Insurance Program, may obtain assistance with payment for physician's services, diagnostic tests, and other outpatient services. Individuals participate voluntarily through enrollment and the payment of a monthly fee.

TERTIARY CARE

Care of a highly technical and specialized nature, provided in a medical center—usually one affiliated with a university—for patients with unusually severe, complex, or unusual disorders. Tertiary care is the highest level of care.

TERTIARY CARE CENTER

A large medical institution, usually a teaching hospital, that provides highly specialized care.

THIRD-PARTY PAYER

An organization, private or public, that pays for or insures at least some of the health care expenses of its beneficiaries. Third-party payers include commercial health insurers, Medicare, and Medicaid.

UNDERWRITING

The process by which an insurer determines whether and on what basis it will accept an application for insurance. Some insurers use medical underwriting to exclude individuals, groups, or coverage for certain health conditions that are expected to incur high costs.

UTILIZATION REVIEW (UR)

The review of services delivered by a health care provider to evaluate the appropriateness, necessity, and quality of the prescribed services. The review can be performed on a prospective, concurrent, or retrospective basis.

Index